PENGUIN BOOKS

SUGAR AND SPICE

Sue Lees was born in India. On leaving school she worked in a refugee camp in Austria, and then trained to be a social worker at Edinburgh University and the London School of Economics. She worked as a probation officer for five years, during which time she took a part-time degree in psychology at Birkbeck College, London. She is author of *Losing Out* (1986) and has published widely in the areas of violence against women, equal opportunities and sexuality. She taught social psychology at Middlesex University, group work at York University and research methods at the University of North London, where she set up one of the first Women's Studies degree courses in 1986. She is now Co-ordinator of the Women's Studies Unit there. Shortly after beginning the research, she suffered a viral illness called Guillam Barree which paralysed her but from which, with the help of her family and friends, she has made a complete recovery. She was joint Chair of the Women's Studies Network (UK) Association from 1989 to 1991 and is the British delegate to the European Women's Studies Research Foundation.

SUE LEES

Sugar and Spice

SEXUALITY AND ADOLESCENT GIRLS

PENGUIN BOOKS

PENGUIN BOOKS

Published by the Penguin Group
Penguin Books Ltd, 27 Wrights Lane, London w8 5tz, England
Penguin Books USA Inc., 375 Hudson Street, New York, New York 10014, USA
Penguin Books Australia Ltd, Ringwood, Victoria, Australia
Penguin Books Canada Ltd, 10 Alcorn Avenue, Toronto, Ontario, Canada m4v 3b2
Penguin Books (NZ) Ltd, 182–190 Wairau Road, Auckland 10, New Zealand

Penguin Books Ltd, Registered Offices: Harmondsworth, Middlesex, England

Published in Penguin Books 1993
10 9 8 7 6 5 4 3 2 1

The moral right of the author has been asserted

Typeset by Datix International Limited, Bungay, Suffolk
Set in 10½/12½ pt Monophoto Baskerville
Printed in England by Clays Ltd, St Ives plc

Contents

Acknowledgements

Many of the ideas in this book have arisen from stormy arguments over a number of years. Without the encouragement of many friends and colleagues and my children, Dan and Jose, this book would not have been possible. I would like to thank in particular Margaret Bluman, Celia Cowie, John Lea, Angela McRobbie, Dave Phillips, Sue Sharpe, Beverley Skeggs, Frank Warner, my sister Diana for giving us a roof above our heads when we were made homeless by the house we live in subsiding, and Dan Lees and Marissa Vernon for transcribing tapes. Lastly I would like to thank all the girls and boys who gave time and enthusiasm to the interviews and group discussions and who have spoken so spontaneously and openly about their lives.

Introduction

Puberty, which gives man the knowledge of greater power, gives to woman the knowledge of her dependence (Tilt 1852:265)

Men and women speak different languages that they assume are the same (Gilligan 1982:173)

As we approach the twenty-first century, one of the greatest problems facing the advanced industrialized countries is the inability of women and men to relate to each other. It is a major source of unhappiness and distress. Violence against women, both in and outside marriage, child sexual abuse, the rising suicide rate among young men, the rise in anorexia and bulimia among adolescent girls, AIDS combined with the soaring divorce rate, all indicate that the institution of the family and the process of child-rearing is in a crisis of transition. Leaving crude indices aside, the difficulty women and men have communicating is expressed in popular films, plays, literature and music, which also show that men's attitudes to women have not kept up with the dramatic changes that have altered women's lives. There are various explanations for why this crisis is occurring. One view is that these changes are brought about by rapid social change in the economy, another attributes the malaise to a breakdown of morality, yet another attributes it to the growing confidence of women to contest their subordination in the family.

Changes in the structure of the economy and social division of labour over the past fifty years have brought about a crisis in gender relations. The old structure of the working-class family established during the nineteenth century, in which the men worked for a 'family wage' while the women managed the home and reared the children, is being rapidly undermined. The decline of older manufacturing industries – a large proportion of whose labour force consisted of unskilled manual labour – has led to rising rates of unemployment for young men. A major factor in this rise has been the removal of unskilled labouring jobs which were the form of entry for young men of the lower working class into the labour force. These were the 'lads' described in Paul Willis's seminal study *Learning to Labour*, a British study written in the 1970s (Willis 1977).

At the same time the proportion of women in the labour force has increased. The growth of flexible, part-time work, much of it low-paid and using new technology, replacing the older manual jobs in a growing service-based economy, and reflecting the expansion until recently in welfare state and public services, has increased employment opportunities for young women. In Britain over the period 1952–92 women have moved from 31 per cent to 45 per cent of the labour force. While the trend to increasing female employment runs in the opposite direction to increasing male unemployment they are, of course, both reflections of a single process of economic change.

These changes in the labour force have naturally been reflected in changes in education. With the introduction of the national curriculum girls and boys now study the same subjects and there is formal commitment to equal opportunities at all levels of education. The expansion of education from the sixties onwards has seen an increasing proportion of girls staying on at school and going into further and higher education. In 1992 for the first time in the UK more young women than young men entered university.

These socio-economic trends form the background to the crisis in gender relations which is the subject matter of this book. As young women stay on longer at school and move increasingly into formerly male preserves of employment it is inevitable that they will begin to question the misogynist attitudes, expectations and behaviour that reflected an older patriarchal social structure in which the man was seen as the family breadwinner and the woman as the subservient home-maker and where women's economic stability lay more in making a 'good' marriage rather than in getting a good job.

For many boys this change represents not simply a move to less stable employment, it means a move to no employment. The old rituals of transition from youth to adulthood marked by leaving school, first employment, joining a stable, male work culture, assisted by older workers – some of whom might be uncles and fathers – integrating into the union, getting married, saving for a first house or flat, have not been re-placed by new ones, they have simply been thrown into crisis by the break in the transition from education to work. Integra-tion has been replaced by marginalization, ambition by frustration.

The sense of frustration is heightened by the mass media, which celebrate for male youth glamour welded to the status symbols of affluence, the trainers, video recorders, leather jackets, motor bikes and cars, all beyond the reach of many young men with no money and no future, who at the same time lack any sense of being part of a whole community suffering collectively as was the case during the Depression or the interwar years. Instead in films and videos young men are presented as violent and are encouraged to emulate toughness, coolness, physical strength and sexual prowess. Desired women are increasingly being represented as a threat to their survival, as violent and vengeful, as for example in the film *Fatal Attraction*. The effect on young men seems to be to lead them to fall back on other ways of asserting their masculinity, on the streets (as in Los Angeles), on the football terraces and in the home by heightened aggressive sexuality and violence. If work no longer brings status, then it will be recovered by violence both to other men and to women. Some young men are genuinely confused as to what is expected of them, yet the new man is more myth than reality. Simultaneously we have a situation where young women are increasingly questioning and rejecting the types of masculinity and femininity that young men are desperately trying to hang on to.

Women's responses to the changing face of femininity are ambivalent and contradictory. On occasion they may connive at their inferiority in order to get along with men, by, for example, playing the 'helpless' female or pretending to be stupid. On the other hand they may subvert the sexism so prevalent in everyday life. The challenging of old stereotypes of male and female behaviour may be a source of unhappiness but also opens up possibilities for transformation.

Until fifteen years ago research on adolescents was almost exclusively concerned with boys. Images of youth that emerged from poetry, literature, psychology, education and sociology were ones of male adolescents or young adults and rarely included girls, let alone focused on them. Experts in child development and sociologists generally assumed that adolescence was similar for girls and boys or that girls were not worth separate consideration. A second weakness was the almost total lack of analysis of gender relations. Rather than examining the savage chauvinism of male youth culture, it has been embraced as a celebration of masculinity. Such studies have accepted sexism uncritically and, by depicting rock bands, drug 'cultures', hippies and even skinheads and other groups romantically, implicitly extolled masculinity. The reason why the day-to-day experience of sexism has been rarely questioned is due to the common sense view of gender divisions as 'natural' and biologically unchangeable. Until the late 1970s, the emphasis was on class differences, with little discussion of gender dominance and subordination, of masculinity and femininity or the effect of these constructions on the development of identity.

This study is not about the area of adolescence that has attracted the most attention. It neither focuses on social problems such as drug addiction, teenage mothers or delinquents, nor is it about the most sophisticated adolescent girls who are involved in media culture. It is instead mainly about ordinary girls, with a smaller sample of boys, both working- and middle-class, some poor, some better off, aged between fifteen and seventeen, living in an inner-city area. In Britain, girls are doing better than boys at school, they are far more visible in public places, in pubs, discos and on the street. The position of young women in the employment market may be weak but some young women have greater access to jobs, albeit low-paid, than young men. Yet at the level of their everyday lived experience, according to my research, their position is one of subordination. They may go to nightclubs or parties but the problem of getting home unscathed is a fear they routinely have to contend with. Girls have to come to grips with daily contradictions to navigate their way through the system of gender domination. The overall effect on girls of this gender oppression is to shake their confidence in themselves and can lead to depression, eating disorders and other disturbances.

My research asks why this process of becoming women and men is not keeping pace with other social changes. We need to explore the meaning of women's and men's worlds if we are to understand the processes by which our identities are constructed. By interviewing adolescents, who are at the critical period of life, when adult identities are shaped and developed, I show how young women and men learn to constitute and reconstitute themselves through social practices in a constantly evolving process and how this process is gendered. Girls and boys learn what behaviour is expected of them, but they do not necessarily accept the demarcation nor does a changing society always provide them with opportunities to fulfil or confirm those expectations.

Our understanding of the world is mediated through language. Words are not simply shapes on a piece of paper, or sounds. Language is intrinsic to the way we make sense of our experiences. Words carry with them a history, in the case of gender, the history of women's relationship to men. Words are also culturally specific. For example, the words man and woman have different meanings in different cultures. Our social relationships, the way girls and boys see each other, are formed through language. It is through language that we express and reinforce power relationships and organize our political and institutional systems. It is through language that we make sense of gender relationships.

There is a large literature on the way language shapes and reflects class (see Labov 1972, Bernstein 1970) and ethnic relationships. Alice Walker in *The Color Purple*, for example, describes how Celie, the main character of the novel, uses black American vernacular English as a means of resistance to oppression and as a way of maintaining racial identity. Similarly I will be claiming that it is through language that gender identities develop, identities that reflect power relationships.

Identity develops, as Simone de Beauvoir (1949, translated 1972) showed, in relation to an 'object' or 'other', and it is by differentiating between women and men that men maintain dominance over women. It is woman who is defined as the object of man's desire.

She is defined and differentiated with reference to man and not he with reference to her, she is the incidental, the inessential as opposed to the essential. He is the subject, he is the Absolute – she is the Other (de Beauvoir 1949, 1972).

Masculinity and femininity do not therefore have some biological 'essence', as is commonly believed, but they are socially constructed through language. There is as much diversity among babies that are allocated to be 'female' as those that are allocated to be 'male'. Some babies are born with a mixture of male and female biological organs and a decision has to be made about how to assign them. Men's domination is not dependent on biology, it is dependent on women's subordination. Masculinity is only meaningful if differentiated from femininity. To maintain dominance it is vital for men that these distinctions are maintained. Deborah Cameron expresses this very clearly:

Nothing is more ridiculous than a woman who imitates a male activity, and is therefore no longer a woman. This can apply not only to speaking and writing, but also to the way a woman looks, the job she does, the way she behaves sexually, the leisure pursuits she engages in, the intellectual activities she prefers and so on *ad infinitum*. Sex differentiation must be rigidly upheld by whatever means are available, for men can be men only if women are unambiguously women (Cameron 1985:155–6).

It is often assumed that words do not have a material effect. 'Sticks and stones may break your bones. But words will never hurt you' goes the old rhyme. But they do. I will show how the use of language, and practices, have material consequences. It is through language that social relationships are daily being shaped, reaffirmed, stabilized and, most importantly, being contested not just at the level of intellectual debate in learned journals but in the daily lives of people. Girls, as we shall see, are limited by the language they have access to, for example in contesting verbal sexual abuse there are very few derogatory words they can use in retaliation to such words as 'whore' and all its synonyms. For a girl to use bad language also carries the risk of being labelled as unfeminine. If they want to describe their sexual organs they only have medical or abusive terms. Yet sexism is being daily contested by many girls and is no longer taken for granted as part of common sense.

I wanted to elicit the terms with which they handle their world, to follow up the meanings through which they relate to that world, meanings both individually held and collectively shared. Like Carol Gilligan, 'the central assumption was that the language [people] use and the connections they make reveal the world that they see and in which they act' (Gilligan, Lyons and Hanmer 1990:2).

The approach taken in this book traverses disciplines. It is an ambitious undertaking, but one that aims to give an overview of the debates that have arisen since girls became the focus of research fifteen years ago. Drawing on my own empirical research on adolescent girls and boys, undertaken in the early and mid 1980s and published in my earlier book, *Losing Out*, I relate my findings to some of the core debates that have framed the question of girls within sociology, psychology, women's studies, and educational studies.

I explore how girls and boys see their lives in their own terms rather than by asking questions about which I have preconceptions. Through interviews and group discussions I have analysed their experiences at the level of language, and shown to what extent they are confirming or contesting the taken-for-granted constructions of masculinity and femininity. I wanted to find out how girls experienced the world, how they saw friendship, school, love and marriage, work and the future. I wanted to hear what they thought when they chatted in groups of friends and talked. In the 1980s a researcher Celia Cowie and I interviewed 100 fifteen- to sixteen-year-old girls at three London schools and thirty boys.[1] We used unstructured interviews and group discussions. All the interviews and group discussions were tape-recorded and later transcribed. The girls and boys who were from varied social class and ethnic groups were interviewed singly, or could choose to bring a friend along. They were also interviewed in groups of three to five friends. The first two schools were mixed: unusually both had women head teachers, who were attempting to put into force an equal opportunities programme. One school was predominantly white, working-class, and the other had a high proportion of different ethnic groups. The third was single-sex with a mainly middle-class intake, which was used to investigate the importance of class differences.

As well as investigating the similarities between girls, I wanted to see in what ways race and class differences were seen as important by girls. Pupils at London schools, where the research was undertaken, came from a range of ethnic backgrounds. Most had been brought up in this country, but many were bilingual – there were girls whose families had come from Greece, different parts of Africa, the Caribbean, India, Pakistan, Bangladesh, Italy, China, Israel, Spain and a couple from Eastern Europe. All the schools were attempting to teach a multi-cultural curriculum and two schools were involved in combating racism. Unfortunately I did not have adequate funding to undertake a detailed analysis of the similarities and differences between all the social groups. From reading the transcripts it was not always possible to say what ethnic background the girl came from, and all girls used similar terms to describe how sexual reputation constrained their lives. Despite quite dramatic cultural and religious differences between girls, they do appear, on the basis of imperfect data, to share some crucial experiences of being girls in Britain, independent of culture.[2]

After interviewing girls, I widened the research to include a smaller sample of boys. Together with Dave Phillips, a male colleague, six group discussions were held composed of about five boys from different ethnic and social backgrounds who also selected which groups to join. Later, some of them were individually interviewed. I wanted to ask boys about gender relations, an area that has been neglected in youth research. The contrast between the girls' and boys' groups was startling. The girls interacted and were introspective, talked about relationships and feelings, worries and concerns. The boys all talked at the same time, interrupted each other, rarely listened to what other boys said and vied for attention and dominance; they were very lively. Controlling the group led by Dave Phillips was a bit like refereeing a football match. I seemed to calm their exuberance and they appeared to talk more seriously and less jokingly, as though there was no need to impress me, perhaps because I was considered less influential than my colleague. Unfortunately we only interviewed one Afro-Caribbean boy, though more participated in the group discussions. Interviewed six boys from Bangladesh. The constitution of masculinity may well show different forms between different nationalities, but it is impossible on the basis of such a small sample to make generalizations. More research is needed in this area.

Five main topics were explored – what girls and boys said about school; friendship with girls and boys; their families; sexuality; and their expectations for the future. The interview technique was non-directive. A central assumption that informed the research was that what girls and boys have to say about their lives is significant and has not previously been heard. The method of interviewing was to ask open-ended questions and then to follow up what the girls and boys said to uncover exactly what they meant. I wanted to elicit the terms with which they handle their world, to follow up the meanings through which they relate to that world, meanings both individually held and collectively shared. Girls were also given a questionnaire about their home circumstances, parental occupations, education, religion and interests, and about the girls' own friendship networks. I invited a group of girls from different class and ethnic groups from the two schools to video two days of group discussions. This was later made into a short film. The video was shown to the girls and they were asked what they thought about it.

Very few comparable studies of girls are available, and researchers have commented on the inaccessibility of girls. These other studies were carried out in youth clubs. By conducting interviews and discussions during school time rather than after I avoided encroaching on the girls' own time and provided a welcome diversion from classes. Girls were not only willing to talk but prepared to discuss intimate questions about their lives with what appeared to be openness and frankness as well as verve and humour. This is not to say that the girls did not view me as different from themselves, and this might have affected their responses. Several commented on my clothes, and others were perplexed that my colleague, Celia Cowie, was not married but had a child. It is impossible to know how far such factors influenced the course of the interviews. We avoided answering personal questions until each interview was over, when we would tell them anything they wanted to know. To divulge personal details during the interview might lead to bias – interviewees often want to please the interviewer and may say what they think she wants to hear. Since we were bringing up very personal issues it was particularly important that the girls should see us as respecting any feelings they expressed, whether they related to aspects of sex, class or race. This research method allowed girls to speak for themselves. Apart from providing a rich source of material, as the discussions did seem to 'take off' when the girls and boys lost their self-consciousness, the groups provided an essential source of information about the contradictions and ambiguities in their views.

Non-directive, semi-structured interviews, as opposed to more formal, quantifiable methods, enable the subjects' responses to be followed up, and allow the subjects to be more specific and more revealing of both intimate material and the connections across material that indicate the social context of those feelings, beliefs and ideas. By focusing on the terms girls used to describe their world, and by looking across at the transcripts, light was thrown on the communalities of the girls' lives and how individual experiences were socially structured.

Given the strictures against the researcher making any positive critical intervention in order to avoid bias, it was difficult at times to know how far to question the girls' ideas. A useful technique was to ask girls to give examples to illustrate exactly what they meant by what they said. So if they referred to the word 'slag',[3] I would question them about when the term might be used or what happened if a boy boasted he had had two girls. Another useful strategy was to ask girls to discuss in a group what a girl's reputation rested on and whether violence ever occurred. Girls often disagreed with each other, and discussions were dynamic and often heated. Girls, for example, had strong views about abortion yet were horrified that a female teacher decided to have a baby on the condition that her husband took on the day-to-day care of the baby as she wanted to continue to work. Girls were on the whole conventional in their attitudes to women's roles and wary of change. My approach could be described as one of conscious partiality (Mies 1983:122), where the researcher identifies her own experience, in this case of the contradictory nature of growing up in a patriarchal society, with girls or women who are the participants.

This is a feminist research project. Initially feminist research was defined as 'research for women, on women and by women', but it was not long before the definition broadened to address not only the question of women's invisibility but also the categories and concepts by which disciplines ordered experience. The language of academia is frequently gender blind. For example, in philosophy 'rationality' is often regarded as a particular male attribute which some philosophers have denied women, arguing that their emotions 'clouded their reason'. 'Work' has been defined by sociologists as 'paid', excluding and marginalizing the domestic and childcare work that all societies allocate to women. Such terms as 'youth' and 'mankind' are used to embrace both girls and boys, women and men, but boys and men are taken as the standard. In youth research, as we shall see, maturity has been defined as the development of autonomy rather than of responsibility for others, or interdependence.

In challenging the taken-for-granted bases of knowledge, feminist research is a subversive activity. It challenges the separation between the public and the private, between reason and emotion, between masculinity and femininity. It is about allowing women's voices to be heard in the curriculum, integrating the study of emotions as well as the study of cognition. It is about radicalizing institutions, modifying their latent and manifest discriminatory policies, changing the face of education. As Bowles and Klein aptly put it in the preface to their book:

It has the potential to alter fundamentally the nature of all knowledge by shifting the focus from androcentricity to a frame of reference in which women's difference and differing ideas, experiences, needs and interests are valid in their own right and form the basis for our teaching and learning (Bowles and Klein 1983:3).

Four core debates about adolescence will be discussed throughout the book. Firstly, the concept of socialization has been criticized as inadequate (Walkerdine 1992). Secondly, one of the main weaknesses of previous research is that the concept of adolescence in so far as girls are concerned, has inappropriately been seen as the development of autonomy. Thirdly, gender is either considered to be irrelevant or sex differences are seen as biologically determined. (At adolescence girls are seen as naturally developing into women and boys into men.) Lastly, that the relations between girls and boys, the constructions of masculinity and femininity that underlie those relations, are not always seen as a reflection of power divisions in a wider society.

The Concept of Socialization

The concept of socialization, the process by which we become women and men, has recently been criticized for failing to take account of social change. It presumes that an established set of relationships exists that children are moulded into, as if these relationships were fixed and unchanging. In other words the assumption is that we develop a firm unchanging sense of self through a process of socialization practices which enables us to undertake our appropriate roles in society. The division between the sexes has been seen as functional for capitalism which, it has been argued, necessitates a clear division between the male 'instrumental' bread-winning role and the female 'emotional' and reproductive role.

By and large socialization theories work with a coherent concept of the adult gender role that in modern societies like our own is not appropriate and can be less convincingly held. In modern life the adult role is fragmented and contradictory. Changes in the economic structure, such as in the decline of heavy industry, have meant that the conventional definition of maleness is losing its force. Physical strength is no longer needed for most work. Likewise the entry of women into the workforce means that the polarity between women and men is now blurred. These traditional adult gender relations may be seen as functionally inappropriate. The loss of traditional masculinity along with loss of job opportunities may be one reason for the rise of the New Right in America (see Weiss 1990).

Bronwyn Davies (1989) argues that the conception of identity in socialization theories is fixed, which precludes any concept of the child as active rather than a passive recipient of socialization.

There is no room in this model of the world for the child as an active agent, the child as theorist, recognizing for him or herself the way the social world is organized. Nor is there acknowledgment of the child as implicated in the construction and maintenance of the social world through the very act of recognizing it and through learning its discursive practices (Davies 1989:5).

Such models are inevitably embedded with sexist assumptions and fail to take into account the contradictory ways in which women and men often behave in different contexts. For example, parents often think they see their adolescent children as undergoing personality changes. But such changes can better be seen as the adolescents 'trying out' different ways of behaviour as part of the process of developing self-knowledge. An alternative theoretical approach is therefore to replace 'personality', as a relatively stable and consistent structure, with 'identity', seen as a mosaic or collage of elements in a contingent relationship with one another. Thus Suzanne Moore argues that 'We can no longer talk of the individual or the self as an autonomous and coherent unity but instead we have to come to understand that we are made up from and live our lives as a mass of contradictory fragments . . .' (Moore 1988:170).

Adolescence and Autonomy

Identity development is very different for a girl than for a boy. While for men identity precedes intimacy and generativity in the optimal cycle of human separation and attachment, for women the tasks of intimacy and identity are fused in such a way that girls come to know themselves through their relationships with others. Gilligan argues that 'male gender identity' is threatened by intimacy, while 'female gender identity' is threatened by separation. Responsibility for others and sensitivity to their needs often conflict with autonomous independent action. Feminists who broke away from the model of femininity that denied female subjectivity and desire, and extolled self-sacrifice, have found it difficult to reconcile the masculine concept of independence with care and concern for others.

Deborah Tannen (1992), Professor of Linguistics at Georgetown University, Washington, DC, comes to remarkably similar conclusions to Carol Gilligan through her analysis of women's and men's conversations. She illustrates how women and men use language in very different ways; women primarily to make connections and reinforce intimacy, men to preserve their independence and negotiate status. This makes it difficult for women and men, and girls and boys, to communicate with each other.

Female adolescence is not then simply about moving from the dependence of childhood to the independence of adult life, as it is with boys. Girls are faced with the problem of how to gain some freedom in a society where caring and dependency are seen as attributes of femininity. They are caught between definitions of femininity and of adolescence (Hudson 1984). The very concept of adolescence is a masculine construct at odds with femininity as constructed in present society. Girls cannot behave like typical adolescents – moodily, recklessly, selfishly rebellious – without infringing the dictates of femininity. To go around looking scruffy renders a girl open to accusations of 'sluttishness'; for a boy torn jeans and a dirty sweatshirt can add to his appeal. But by conforming to models of correct femininity, girls do not escape criticism, nor is this a solution: they are seen as old-fashioned, straight and dull. Girls tread a very narrow line: they mustn't end up being called a slag, but equally they don't want to be thought unapproachable, sexually cold – a tight bitch. Research has shown, for example, that women who conform to cultural stereotypes of female passivity, conformity, lower achievement motivation and vulnerability are likely to be defined as psychologically unhealthy. Women who reject such stereotypes are also likely to be labelled deviant or, if successful in their careers, to be considered 'masculine'.

Education involves a basic contradiction for girls. Being academically successful involves taking on, in so far as they are permitted to, attributes that are considered to be masculine. This can only be achieved at some cost, by behaving in an 'asexual' way. This is similar for girls who enter non-traditional masculine areas such as painting and decorating in youth training schemes, as so graphically described by Anne Stafford (Stafford 1991). Their position in this 'masculine' world is always precarious, which is why so few women have the confidence to speak out and challenge the patriarchal structure of education. Similarly, boys who develop 'feminine' qualities of care and concern for others are seen as 'wimps', unacceptable to the 'macho' culture.

Yet there are far less conflictual models for boys to aspire to. A boy can be confident in his body, which is not blazoned naked on billboards and the subject of critical and often salacious gaze. He may have to take care to avoid gangs of boys but he can enter the public sphere on his own with confidence that he will not be continually sexually harassed. However insecure, a boy can be confident in his superiority to girls. Barbara Hudson argues that much behaviour is legitimated by discourses of adolescence which allow adolescent boys space for experimentation, but no such leeway is given to girls, who are always seen as embryo women, never a developing person (Hudson 1984). Both girls and boys see considerable advantages in being a boy in terms of their greater autonomy, their lack of responsibilities and the double standard of morality.

Much theorizing about identity has overlooked the contradictions of female identity. Erikson, whose model of behaviour is entirely male, sees the concept of identity formation as central to adolescent development (Erikson 1968). He sees the main task of adolescence as the need to develop a sense of self, to verify an identity that can span the discontinuity of puberty and make possible the adult capacity to love and work. Yet his model makes no distinction between the way a girl and a boy face this task. No attention is given to the way female identity rests to such an extent on sexual status and reputation. Gaining an identity as a young girl involves forming an identity – a firm sense of self – in opposition to the depiction of girls as sex objects, in opposition to the characterization of women as no more than sexual beings. For some Asian girls the effect of sexual reputation on their emerging identity can be even more dramatic. It can control everything they do (Wilson 1978).

Biological Essentialism

There is a third respect in which existing theories give an inaccurate perception of how identities are developed. The assumption of a biological basis of difference is being contested also on the basis of evidence from developments in biology itself. Biologists increasingly reject the common sense idea that there is a necessary link between genetic, hormonal and genital sex, that sex differences are to some degree biologically based. Evidence for this derives from studies of children who are misassigned as girls at birth because they are born without external genitals (Kessler and McKenna 1978). Such children have to be reassigned after the late development of external male genitalia at the age of eighteen months or two years and experience great trauma. If biology was important then you would expect their reassignment to be a relief. There are also people who begin life as females and develop male genitalia around puberty (Crapo 1985). The idea that the world can 'be simply divided into bipolar opposites has no more basis than the conceptual division of the world into stupid and intelligent people, or short and tall or beautiful and ugly' (see Davies 1989).

Nor is there any reason why maleness necessarily implies sexual dominance. The female could just as easily be constructed as active and dominant. Bob Connell, an Australian sociologist, points out that it is not

biologically decreed, by the architecture of the genitals, that man must thrust and woman lie still (though that is a belief on which a great tower of sub-Freudian bullshit has been erected, even by otherwise perceptive psychoanalysts). This too is constructed, as a relation, in a practice of sexual encounter that begins with erection and ends with ejaculation, and in which woman's pleasure is marginal to what the man does, or is assumed to be guaranteed by powerful ejaculation. In eroticism focused on the penis and penetration, passive or gentle contact is likely to be dispensed with or hurried through, for fear of losing the erection, failing; and the man may be quite unable to climax except with moving, thrusting (Connell 1983:24).

Power Relations

The last limitation of many previous studies of adolescence is the absence of analysis of the relation of theories of socialization to relations of power within society. As Walkerdine (1990) argues: 'Power is implicated in the power/knowledge relations investigated in the creation and regulation of practices ... Power is shifting and fragmentary, relating to positionings given in the apparatuses of regulation themselves.'

Relations of power are embedded in constructions of masculinity and femininity which underpin the idea of rationality and are central to the process of schooling and to the division between the public and the private sphere – which according to Chodorow (1978) explains the different outcomes of socialization for girls and boys. Drawing on anthropology (see Mead 1949, Rosaldo 1980) she argues that in all societies where women are relegated to the private sphere of domestic and childcare work, they are rendered socially and politically subordinate to men in the public sphere. This is more marked in advanced capitalist societies.

There are problems with reducing woman's subordination to either her role in the family (the private sphere) or in the labour market and public life (the public sphere). First, why are women in an inferior position in the private sphere? It is one thing to find economic or other reasons why women spend the bulk of their lives in the private domain, but this does not of itself explain why their position in that sphere should be one of subordination to men (see Harris 1979). Equally, to show that the roles and activities of the private sphere are predominantly organized around reproduction and childcare is not to explain why men exercise control over women. Such domination cannot be explained simply by reference to men's greater freedom to participate in the public sphere and hence their absence from the private. For why should absence lead to domination? Anthropologists such as Harris (1979) and Rosaldo (1980) cite many examples of cultures in which male supremacy is retained despite the considerable, and at times equal, participation of women and men.

Secondly, explanations that separate the public and private spheres often amount to tautologies. Whatever women do (and their roles vary between societies and through time) tends to become assimilated to the category of 'domestic labour'. Various types of work such as making tea, cleaning up, typing, etc. tend to be characterized as 'women's work', whether they are done at home or in the office or works canteen.

The analysis used in this book attempts to overcome these

problems by focusing on language as a form of activity or material practice in itself – the analysis of language is in a position to grasp the dynamics of female subordination to men not in terms of, but rather irrespective of, the separation between the public and private spheres. The discussion of power does not relate to whether girls are concentrated in certain roles rather than others, but can be seen as a field of force in which girls and boys are equally trapped, rather than being exercised by boys over girls. Thus it is less important to show that boys use a different language to abuse others, than to realize that whoever is talking, virtually all the terms of abuse available are ones that denigrate women. Girls use the same derogatory terms as boys.

This language plays a crucial role in the constitution of male relationships both inside and outside the home. As Cynthia Cockburn describes in her account of male compositors:

Many women who have had reason to work with compositors will confirm my experience that they make a big show of apologizing for 'bad language' that would offend a woman's ears. By this they don't mean the odd 'damn' or 'bloody'. The social currency of the compositing room is woman and women objectifying talk, from sexual expletives and innuendo through to narration of exploits or fantasies. The wall is graced with four-colour litho 'tits' and 'bums'. Even the computer is used to produce life-size print-outs of naked women (Cockburn 1983).

We need to understand the way in which social practices and systems of representation operate and appear to work without any direct coercion. In order to grasp how the cultural codes of behaviour are understood and are effective at defining sex roles, we need to examine what passes as 'common sense'. We need to examine such assumptions as: it is natural for boys to be after one thing in their relationships with girls and that a boy needs sex while girls do not and that it is quite all right for him to cajole girls into bed. To initiate sex is seen as unfeminine yet at the same time girls are seen as responsible for boys' sexual urges. Girls 'ask for it' and a girl has only herself to blame if ultimately an encounter with a boy results in rape. To rebuff boys or take little interest in them is then to be unnatural.

Through the voices of ordinary girls and boys I will indicate how the politics of everyday life is being constantly debated and worked out. Female adolescence is an experience where girls are daily confronted with contradictions that they have to develop strategies to deal with. I debate the way masculinities and femininities are constructed and lived out by the girls and boys, and how they see themselves in relation to those constructs. This is not to dismiss economic and structural determinants. It is a dynamic and political approach. Whereas there might well exist structural forces which in the last instance can explain behaviour, to the extent to which this process takes place mainly through language, it is accessible to consciousness and therefore can and is being changed. It raises the possibility that by becoming aware of these processes that constrain communication between girls and boys, more meaningful reciprocal relationships can develop.

Chapter 1

This chapter focuses on the way girls and boys are preoccupied in their talk about sexuality. Girls are aware of the injustice of the way they are treated by boys and how they are seen in terms of their sexual reputation. Contrary to popular belief, the most prevalent form of abuse, 'slag', which is commonly understood to mean a girl who sleeps around promiscuously or is a 'whore', often bears no relation to a girl's actual sexual behaviour. It can just as easily be applied to a girl who dresses, talks or behaves in a certain way. The only constraint on the use of 'slag' is its application to a girl who has no steady boyfriend. The chapter will explore the ways in which this leads to and reproduces a girl's subordination and shows how sexual abuse functions to maintain male solidarity and confirm the power of masculinity. The way sexual and racial stereotypes, though not identical, are in some respects similar to each other will be explored.

Chapter 2

The second chapter looks at the social relations between girls and boys, at different ethnic and class groups, and shows how girls and boys live in different social worlds. The ambiguities and contradictions girls face in maintaining friendships in the context of defending their reputations are outlined. This study refutes the common portrayal of girls as confined to a 'bedroom culture'. Many girls do have wide friendship networks. However girls' friendships are limited by the different terms in which they enter the public sphere – of sport, music, entertainment and social activities.

Chapter 3

The rising divorce rate and increase in cohabitation suggest that girls see marriage more realistically and less romantically than in the past. This chapter deals with the contradiction between the unromantic and stark picture of marriage that emerges from the girls' descriptions and their commitment – if somewhat resigned – to the idea of marriage, or cohabitation leading to marriage. The apparent contradictions between wanting to get married and postponing it, wanting a career yet failing to pursue the appropriate qualifications and wanting to have children but seeing the isolation of mothers with children around them will be explored. The strategy most girls adopt is to postpone this predicament for as long as possible, or for at least ten years. Four strategies that girls adopt to deal with this contradiction will be discussed.

Chapter 4

It is often assumed that the educational system is impartial between girls and boys, and that the experience of school is the same for both sexes. This chapter uncovers a different reality. It shows how education perpetuates and reinforces sexual divisions. This disadvantages boys in relation to their family responsibilities and girls in terms of their academic development. Girls' responses to schooling are contradictory. Many now progress to higher education, yet even then research suggests that the majority give priority to their boyfriends' or husbands' careers and give up their own aspirations. A model of education is advocated which involves creating collective practices to counter gender domination. A model of education is proposed that integrates the need to develop caring and responsible human beings as well as rational abilities.

Chapter 5

This chapter puts forward a feminist approach to sex education. Sexuality is silenced and stifled in the education system. Though every interaction is laced with sexual innuendo, sexual relations are barely mentioned and have only recently begun to be questioned. In this context sex education has been negligible. In the present climate in Britain, with increasing administrative control over the curriculum – such as Clause 28 which forbids the discussion of lesbianism and homosexuality – the movement towards quantifiable results and standardized testing, the lack of flexibility in most school structures and the low status of teachers, everything militates against the approach I am advocating. Teachers are faced with greater constraints, from parents, from managers and from the curriculum, than in the early 1970s. This leaves little space for schools to be 'public sites for the discourse of possibility', where students would be empowered to examine their lives critically.

Chapter 6

Violence experienced by girls within sexual relationships, and bullying which often involves attacks on sexual reputation, leads to low self-esteem, depression and can result in suicide. This chapter discusses the place of violence in the girls' and boys' lives.

For working-class boys in particular, physical violence is presented as a legitimate way of gaining male status. Violence is often sparked off by taunts about sexual reputation, and is seen as a way of defending the 'good' woman from sexual approaches. For girls male violence is often seen as natural. I show how girls often absolve boys of responsibility for violent behaviour. Gender differences in the development of morality are discussed in relation to the work of Carol Gilligan.

Chapter 7

Different strategies girls use to pave a way through this labyrinth of harassment are identified. Since their whole lives are circumscribed by the constraints of male taunts, girls have to develop ways of coping and resisting. Various tactics adopted, some more successful than others, can be broadly categorized as leading to conformity, avoidance or resistance. It appears to be very difficult for girls to organize collectively against boys. Gender is not simply reproduced. Girls' reactions to these processes of subordination are contradictory, but boys' sexism is being daily contested in a way that would have been unthinkable fifteen years ago.

Chapter 8

The last chapter reformulates the meaning of autonomy and dependence to encompass the interdependence of women and men. Different ways of transforming gender relations are put forward. This involves the creation of a morality of responsibility for caring which would enable both girls and boys to develop their potentialities in the twenty-first century and move forward to a world where women will be valued for their contribution both to the home and paid work and where men will take on equal responsibility for domesticity and raising children.

I am grateful to the now-abolished Inner London Education

Authority and to my own institution, the University of North London, who funded the research, and to the Nuffield Foundation, from which charitable funding body I obtained a small grant, and to the many others who have spent countless hours in discussion.

Notes

1. The research and early work was carried out with Celia Cowie.
2. One proviso should however be made. Being a white researcher may have meant that some girls were unwilling fully to divulge their experiences. They may have been reluctant to talk to a white woman and criticize anything that happens in their community to outsiders. I may also have not been sufficiently sensitive to ask the most appropriate questions. In the group discussions however girls often seemed to forget that I was there and many of the discussions took off and became very animated.
3. 'Slag', according to Jane Mills, entered the English language in the mid-sixteenth century, to denote a piece of refuse matter separated from a metal in the process of smelting. By the end of the eighteenth century the sense of waste in 'slag' became combined with the word 'slack', which developed from the old English word denoting indolent, careless or remiss, to mean loose. The word 'slut' denotes laziness, untidiness and dirt as much as promiscuity.

Bibliography

Beauvoir, S. de, 1972, *The Second Sex*, translated by H. M. Parshley, Penguin Books

Bernstein, B., 1970, *Class Codes and Control*, Routledge and Kegan Paul

Bowles, G., and Klein, R., 1983, *Theories of Women's Studies*, Routledge and Kegan Paul

Cameron, D., 1985, *Feminism and Linguistic Theory*, Macmillan

Chodorow, N., 1978, *The Reproduction of Mothering: Psychoanalysis and the Sociology of Gender*, University of California Press

Cockburn, C., 1983, *Brothers: Male Dominance and Technological Change*, Pluto

Connell, R. W., 1983, *Which Way is Up? Essays on Class, Sex and Culture*, Allen and Unwin

Crapo, L., 1985, *Hormones: The Messengers of Life*, Freeman & Co.

Davies, B., 1989, *Frogs and Snails and Feminist Tales*, Allen and Unwin

Erikson, E., 1968, *Identity, Youth and Crisis*, New York, Norton

Gilligan, C., 1982, *In a Different Voice*, Harvard University Press

Gilligan, C., Lyons, N., and Hanmer, T., 1990, *Making Connections: The Relational Worlds of Adolescent Girls at Emma Willard School*, Cambridge, Harvard University Press

Harris, O., 1979, 'Households as Natural Units', in Young, K., Wolkowitz, C., and McCullagh, R. (eds.), *Of Marriage and the Market*, CSE Books

Hudson, B., 1984, 'Femininity and Adolescence', in McRobbie, A., and Nava, M., *Gender and Generation*, Macmillan

Kessler, S., and McKenna, W., 1978, *Gender: An Ethnomethodological Approach*, University of Chicago Press

Labov, W., 1972, *Sociolinguistic Patterns*, University of Pennsylvania Press

Mead, M., 1949, *Male and Female*, Dell Publication

Mies, M., 1983, 'Toward a Methodology for Feminist Research', in Bowles, G., and Klein, R., *Theories of Women's Studies*, Routledge and Kegan Paul

Moore, S., 1988, 'Getting a Bit of the Other – the Pimps of Post-modernism', in Chapman, R., and Rutherford, J. (eds.), *Male Order: Unwrapping Masculinity*, Lawrence and Wishart

Rosaldo, M., 1980, 'The Use and Abuse of Anthropology: Reflections on Feminism and Cross-Cultural Understanding', in *Signs* 5, No. 3

Stafford, A., 1991, *Trying Work*, Edinburgh University Press

Tannen, D., 1992, *You Just Don't Understand: Women and Men in Conversation*, Virago

Tilt, E., 1852, *The Elements of Health, and Principles of Feminine Hygiene*, Henry Bohen

Walkerdine, V., 1990, *Schoolgirl Fictions*, Verso

Walkerdine, V., 1992, 'Girlhood Through the Looking-Glass', plenary paper at the Alice in Wonderland Conference, Amsterdam, June 1992

Weiss, L., 1990, *Working Class Without Work: High School Students in a Deindustrialized Economy*, Routledge, Chapman and Hall

Willis, P., 1977, *Learning to Labour*, Saxon House

Wilson, A., 1978, *Finding a Voice*, Virago

Chapter 1
The Structure of Sexual Relations

I contend that the original loose woman is the free woman – loose and free from bonds and bondage to men. The loose woman is the unattached woman. And because she resisted attachment to men, she became deprived not only of patriarchal protection but of patriarchal repute (Raymond 1991:64)

It's a vicious circle. If you don't like them, then they'll call you a tight bitch. If you go with them they'll call you a slag afterwards (Helen, aged sixteen)

Only in the last fifteen years or so have adolescent girls been the focus of studies, and we still do not know a great deal about how girls experience life in what is often depicted as the turbulent period of adolescence.[1] Myths abound – about the outbreak of adolescent promiscuity heralded by the availability of the pill and greater freedom, about the problem of teenage pregnancy and girls who are 'beyond control' of their parents, about epidemics of anorexia, bulimia and now AIDS, rave parties and the 'breakdown' of the family. Though these media scandals are exaggerated, change is underway, but by no means in one direction. At sixteen, though girls in my research are freer in some respects than previous generations, they are aware that they get a raw deal, are subjected to verbal abuse and some are already burdened with domestic chores. For many girls, by adolescence they are already locked into a life centred on domesticity, subservience, subordination and motherhood, any career aspirations or personal ambition or freedom holding second place to the ideal of finding the man of their dreams. Whether girls are successful in resisting such a fate is an open question. Many accept the difference between girls and boys as biological. Others question the traditional female role, and feminism is part of their agenda. At sixteen, though many boys may still treat girls as inferior, they are also aware of feminism in a way that would have been unthinkable fifteen years ago.

In this chapter I investigate the barriers to equality and locate them primarily in practices underlying the social relations between girls and boys, practices that are often blatantly sexist. I was astonished at the prevalence of verbal sexist abuse in daily use among adolescents. The vocabulary is prolific – slag, slut, tart, whore, cow, dog, bitch, pricktease, crumpet, skirt, flash, nympho, ass, tail, easy lay, scrubber, good screw, dirty ticket to name but a few of the terms used. Dale Spender (1980) in *Man Made Language* reports a study undertaken by Julia Stanley of words used to describe women and found that far more of these referred to sexual behaviour than for men. She uncovered 220 words which referred to the sexually promiscuous female and only twenty to a sexually promiscuous male. This chapter aims to make girls' experience visible, to take what girls say seriously and to analyse the ways girls both conform and resist (or subvert) the sexism around them. It gradually emerged that all girls, regardless of differences in class, income, intelligence or ethnic group, were concerned and anxious about their sexual reputation. I also consider the relation of racist and sexist stereotyping.

In the eighties women have spoken out about child sexual abuse, sexual harassment and date rape as never before. Girls have higher aspirations and greater confidence and are starting to appear however marginally in more positive roles in the music industry, in fiction and in the public arena. Issues of sexual orientation and female sexual pleasure are on the agenda. Why therefore do so many girls continue to accept their subordination and not collectively resist domination by boys? The girls I interviewed did not view the future optimistically or romantically but with a realism about women's lives, laden with fatalism. As one girl entreated after I had given a talk at her school, 'We know it is unfair, but what can we do about it?'

As girls approach adolescence they experience a drop in self-confidence. An American psychologist, Emily Hancock, in her Harvard case study of twenty women, identifies a turning point in a girl's life – the period between the ages of eight and ten – when she crystallizes a distinct and vital sense of self that she then loses in the process of growing up female. Women, Hancock argues, 'learn to think of themselves as flawed and unacceptable and so become uncertain, unfulfilled, anxious, depressed and despairing' (Hancock 1990). How is such malignant nonsense learned and can it be unlearned and a child's original self-acceptance found again? British researchers too have found that between the ages of thirteen and sixteen some girls in schools lose confidence, become more passive, contribute less in class and become less eager to participate (Spender and Sarah 1980, Spender 1982). In this chapter I show how girls lose confidence because their identity rests to such an extent on their sexual reputation, which is precarious and crucial to them.[2]

Girls walk a narrow line: they must not be seen as too tight, nor as too loose. Girls are preoccupied in their talk with sexuality, and in particular with the injustice of the way in which they are treated by boys. Defining girls in terms of their sexuality rather than their attributes and potentialities is a crucial mechanism of ensuring their subordination to boys. 'Nice girls don't' is a phrase all girls understand, even if standards of sexual morality are more liberal. The terms of abuse are so taken for granted that girls do not question them and are themselves drawn into judging other girls in terms of their reputation. One reason for this is that to mix with girls whose reputation is suspect can be 'contaminating' to one's own reputation. The only security girls have against bad reputations is to confine themselves to the 'protection' of one partner. Yet such a resolution involves dependency and loss of autonomy precisely because women's position in the family is subordinate and unequal.

Girls and boys talk about sexuality in quite different ways.

For boys respectability is not crucial. On the contrary, their sexual reputation is enhanced by varied experience: bragging to other boys about how many girls they have 'made'. As Jacky, a working-class sixteen-year-old, and Leiser, a middle-class eighteen-year-old girl, described:

> A boy can be called a stud and people like and respect him – they have no responsibilities, they can just be doing what they want and if they are called a stud then they think it's good, they think it's a compliment . . . It's a sort of status symbol. (Jacky)

> I think it's made a sin for women to enjoy sex. From the time we begin enjoying sex we're called slags, or we can't have too many friends that are men. The ones who have good rapport with boys are called slags and the ones who don't are simply called tight bitches. 'Never get close to her', y'know, 'prude', and I don't think it ever stops. (Leiser)

A boy boasts about sex, but a girl is desperate to keep it quiet: her reputation is under threat, not merely if she is known to have sex (except with a steady) but for a whole range of behaviour often quite unconnected with sex. This is because she is always seen in terms of her sexuality, subjected to verbal and sometimes physical sexual abuse. For a boy, reputation depends on many other things, like being tough, witty, smart or good at sports. His standing in the world is not only determined by his sexual status or conquests. Equally important is his sporting or fighting prowess, his ability to 'take the mickey' or be one of the boys. As Paul Willis comments in *Learning to Labour*:

It is the capacity to fight which settles the final pecking order. It is not often tested ability to fight which valorizes status based usually and interestingly on other grounds: masculine presence, being from a famous family, being funny, being good at 'blagging', extensiveness of informal contacts (Willis 1977).

For a girl it is the defence of her sexual reputation that

determines her standing with girls and boys, certainly around the age of fifteen or so. The emphasis on assumed sexual experience to a girl's reputation is shown by a whole battery of insults that are in everyday use among young people. The effect of this verbal abuse is to silence girls, to make it difficult for them to discuss their sexual desires and to throw each girl back on her own resources to protect her reputation. For boys, talking about sex, whether bragging or putting down girls, enhances camaraderie among them. Their experience is voiced, yet it is a distorted form of experience. Pressure is on them to boast about their conquests, about domination and perform-ance, not about how close they felt to a girl and how well they got on with each other.

Sexism appears to be an important feature of male bonding, where denigration of girls and women is a crucial ingredient of camaraderie in male circles. The masculine tradition of drink-ing and making coarse jokes usually focuses on the 'dumb sex object', 'the nagging wife' or, more derogatively, 'horny dogs' and 'filthy whores'. Learning to be masculine invariably entails learning to be sexist: being a bit of a lad and being con-temptuous of women just go 'naturally' together. Paul Willis in his study of working-class boys talks of boys' relations to girls as 'Exploitative and hypocritical. Girls are pursued, some-times roughly, for their sexual favours, often dropped and labelled "loose" when they give in' (Willis 1977:67).

The asymmetry between girls and boys is illustrated by the term 'slag', which can be used in a whole range of circum-stances. It implies that a girl sleeps around, but this may in fact have nothing to do with the case in point. A girl can be referred to as a slag if her clothes are too tight, too short, too smart or in any way sexually provocative, if she hangs about with boys, is she talks to another girl's boyfriend, if she talks too loudly or too much. It is an ever-present threat; a mecha-nism whereby boys can control girls' behaviour, whether sexual or otherwise, although no equivalent term exists for boys. Any girl is in danger from the 'slag' label at any time, and the girls agreed that the one way to redeem yourself is to get a steady boyfriend. For a girl to admit to feelings of sexual desire is a transgression of this code and can lead to a sullied reputation.

In the media, paradoxically, a girl's body is salaciously discussed, displayed naked on billboards, desired and denigrated. A man's body is concealed and it is even against the law to portray an erect penis publicly. Learning to be a girl, therefore, involves learning to conform to, resist and somehow survive the blatant sexism all around and to be reticent about your own desires. Camaraderie among girls is rarely enhanced by sexist talk as there is no vocabulary of abuse to level at boys. Criticizing the sexism of boys labels a girl a man-hater or a lesbian. It in no way enhances femininity. Quite the contrary. Girls who contest the unfair subordination of girls are likely to be regarded as show-offs or lesbians. There is no commonly used equivalent to the word misogynist, a man who hates women.

Amrit Wilson (1978) who undertook the first British study of Asian girls in the late 1970s described how in conversations she had with girls from many language groups and religions, in every part of Britain, 'reputation came up all the time'. It was not just important but was the 'bane of their lives from adolescence to the early years of marriage. It controls everything they do and adds a very tangible danger to any unconventional action' (Wilson 1978:102). Girls as young as twelve are frightened to go out with boys as they are afraid of the reputation they would get. Sofia, a Muslim girl of nineteen, described how if you go out with a man in Southall

> He will go around and boast to his friends that he's been out with this girl and he's done this to her and that to her. Even if he hasn't, he'll boast about it. Then they get the girl's name bad. That's why girls try and keep it quiet when they're going out with a bloke, because they don't want anyone to know. It's quite different

for boys. They can get away with it. Their names can't ever get spoilt.

Reputation is a conservative force controlling everything in Asian societies, as male pride, or *izzat*, depends on it. Disgracing your family means harming the family *izzat*. A girl's family can be disgraced by the clothes she wears, the way she talks, where she is seen and all the various indicators of a girl's reputation, indeed any indication that she is independent. Some girls do take risks and go out with boys. Asian families do vary. Some Asian girls and women have argued that they do not experience lack of freedom in not leaving their families and communities. They affirm their need to be free within the family and criticize specific aspects of their cultures, including particular kinds of arranged marriages, but they also recognize that the black family, like the working-class family, can be a bastion of defence against class or racial oppression (Amos and Parmar 1987, Brah and Minhas 1985). There is no clear basis for inferring that Asian girls are more oppressed than white girls.

What is the meaning of sexist language for boys and men and why does it depend to such an extent on denigrating women? It is the means of maintaining power over girls and women. Achieving manhood involves a permanent process of struggle and confirmation. Madeleine Arnot (1982) sees this as a dual process of men distancing women and femininity from themselves and maintaining the hierarchy and social superiority of masculinity by devaluing the female world. Calling girls slags accomplishes exactly these two processes. It both distances boys from girls and keeps girls in control. To be a real man, to grow to manhood, involves differentiating oneself from all that is female. Boys therefore abuse each other by using words such as 'woman' or 'motherfucker', and even 'poof', words denoting femininity, to gain solidarity with each other.

How girls and boys develop a gendered subjectivity is dependent on this language. As Bronwyn Davies outlines,

In learning the language [children] learn to constitute themselves
and others, as unitary beings, as capable of coherent thought, as
gendered and as one who is in a particular relation to others.
Language is both a resource and a constraint. It makes social
personal being possible but it also limits the available forms of being
to those which make sense within the terms of the language provided
(Davies 1989).

This view is dynamic. Society is undergoing constant
change. Both girls and boys are continuously structured and
restructuring themselves through language. In this way language has a material existence. It defines our possibilities and
limitations, it constitutes our subjectivities (Black and Coward
1981). The effects of sexist language are as significant in
relation to the structuring of boys' identities as of girls'.
Masculinity and femininity can only be seen as complementary. As Bob Connell, who has tried to come to grips with the
problem of masculinity, comments: 'Masculinity never exists
by itself. It exists in relation to femininity, in the context of an
over-arching structure of gender relations' (Connell, Radican
and Martin 1987:6).

The Vocabulary of Abuse

The vocabulary of abuse raises many questions about the
construction of sexuality, the place of love and marriage in the
girls' lives and the social organization of gender relations. The
commonest insult, used by both sexes, is 'slag', which arose
spontaneously and vividly in all the groups I interviewed and
took me by surprise, since it is almost entirely neglected in the
literature on youth. But almost all the insults in frequent use
seem to relate to a girl's sexual reputation. It is crucial to note
that the insults might bear no relation to a girl's actual sexual
behaviour. But this does not make things any easier for the
girls: an unjustified tag can stick as easily as a justified one.
Different words carry varying degrees of opprobrium or dis-
repute. They could be used in a light-hearted way or more

aggressively. Some of the words are animalistic: bird and kitten can be used affectionately, but dog, bitch, cow are used abusively, though they are less threatening than slag (or its somewhat worse equivalent, slut). Lisa, a girl in my research, makes a distinction between the animalistic names and the more derogatory:

> You can be called bitch, slag, slut . . . I wouldn't like to be called some of them, but I don't mind being called a cow.

When asked the difference she replied:

> Well, it's probably that they all mean the same thing, but you can say it in a nice way or you can say it in a horrible way. Like, of all of them I wouldn't want to be called a slut. If you're called a cow or a blind dog or something like that – a cow or a dog – you know it as well, 'cos they can see it. But when someone calls you a slut or a slag they could be one, 'cos why has the other person called her a slag or a slut? It's probably because they are one.

What is a Slag?

The term 'slag' and its equivalents – slut, scrubber, old dog, easy lay – are frequently mentioned in the various books written about boys but have received little serious analysis as a cultural form: 'Certainly reputations for "easiness" – deserved or not – spread very quickly. The lads are after the "easy lay" at dances, though they think twice about being seen to "go out" with them' (Willis 1977:44).

It has been taken for granted that everyone knows what the term refers to. It has been assumed that the terms 'slag' or 'easy lay' simply apply to certain identifiable girls. But as soon as you raise doubts about the deservedness of the reputation 'easy', and more especially when you ask girls to whom and how the terms are applied, it becomes clear that you have only begun to scratch the surface of a very complex phenomenon. While everyone apparently knows 'a slag' and stereotypically depicts her as thick, untidy, untastefully dressed and made-up, loud-mouthed and, of course, as someone who sleeps around, it seems that such a stereotype bears no relation to the girls (virtually any girls) to whom the term is applied. Paradoxically it seems to be the 'pretty' girl who is most likely to be designated a slag, not the unattractive girl who is categorized as 'too tight' or 'a dog'. One proviso should perhaps be mentioned. Girls and boys at this age live in close communities and the gossip and innuendo may be particularly strong in such contexts. Reputation continues to be crucial but girls who move away from home are protected to some degree by anonymity, at least in big cities.

The first thing that is striking about the use of the term 'slag' is the difficulty of getting any clear definition of what it implies from those who use it. This is true for girls and boys. Take Sadie's description of what she calls a 'proper slag':

I do know one or two slags. I must admit they're not proper slags.

Q *Can you describe what a proper slag is?*

Available aren't they? Just like Jenny, always on the look-out for boys, non-stop. You may not know her but you always see her and every time you see her she's got a different fella with her, you get to think she's a slag. Don't you? She's got a different fella every minute of the day.

Q *So it is just talking to different boys?*

You see them, some of them, they look as innocent as anything, but I know what they're like.

There are two conclusions that can be drawn. Firstly, though the implication here is that the girl who is called a 'slag' sleeps around, this is by no means clear. Everyone apparently knows a slag and stereotypes her as someone who sleeps around, but in reality the insult often bears no relation at all to a girl's actual sexual behaviour. Secondly and following from this, any girl, particularly if she does not have a boyfriend, if she is as the girls termed it 'unattached', has to be constantly aware that the category 'slag' may be applied to her. And there is no hard and fast distinction between the categories, since the status is always disputable, the gossip often unreliable, the criteria obscure.

The implication is that all kinds of social behaviour have a potential sexual significance if the girl is available – and even the term 'available' is two edged, as any girl who is not bound up in a relationship with one man is supposedly potentially available. It shows that women are always defined in relation to men, whether they want to be or not.

The most pernicious ploy in the girl's eyes is when boys make up that they have slept with a girl and then spread around that she is a 'slag'. This is what Lesley, a black girl, referred to as a 'boy's mouthing':

> Oh, I've slept with someone, I done this, I done that and it's not true. When something's not true, that's the worst, because if it's true fair enough – though he shouldn't say nothing – if he's so immature he has to go boasting about it. But to lie about it, that's the worst. If they don't get what they want they lie about it anyway. That to me – that's stupid.

Karen, a white girl, out most nights at discos with a wide circle of friends, sums it up:

> Boys are boys and if they don't get what they want, they're going to lie about it anyway, 'cos they're show-offs. If a boy takes you out or boasts that he has slept with more than one girl, his reputation is enhanced.

They both agreed that if a boy tells his mates that he's been with three different girls, his mates would all say: 'Oh, lucky you,' or, 'Well done my son, you're a man.' The pressure is on boys to boast about their sexual conquests. They have to act big in front of their friends. As Sasha explained:

> They might say, 'Oh, I've had her.' Then it starts spreading round. She might be really quiet or something and they'll say, 'Oh, she's not quiet when you get outside the school.' Someone else will take it in the wrong way and it'll carry on from there.

No wonder that girls always fear boys going behind their backs and saying: 'Oh, you know, I had it with her.' It is the girl's morality that is always under the microscope, whereas anything the boy does is all right.

Boys, unlike the girls, generally supported the idea of a double standard. Jim, a fifteen-year-old boy, thought a boy should have experience before marriage but not a girl:

> It's ridiculous for a girl. Going out with too many boys. They've still got to get married.

I asked Assad, an Asian boy, whether he thought the double standard was still strong. He replied:

> Yeah, if a boy goes out with lots of girls then he'll think he's OK, but if a girl goes out with lots of boys it's not OK. It's a bit old fashioned.
>
> Q *Why isn't it OK if a girl goes out with lots of boys?*
>
> People don't think it's OK. They think she should stay at home, be a wife all day long.

These comments are somewhat hesitant, and the boys realize that the double standard is not fair. This may indicate a subtle shift in social attitudes or imply that they are reticent about admitting their sexism to a female researcher.

A number of girls described girls who had not slept around but had been out with a number of different boys in a short period because they were unlucky enough to be dropped by a number of boys. This led people to start saying, 'Oh God, who is she with tonight?' This distinction pinpoints what is really biting about being called a slag: that any girl is open to being categorized as one – any girl could be one.

Girls do not all react similarly to such abuse, but all girls have to develop strategies for dealing with it, as we shall see in the chapter on strategies of coping and resistance. Some girls laugh the insults off, others feel threatened, afraid or upset. But regardless of whether or not the accusations are justified, few girls feel able simply to ignore them or to resist them effectively – to give as good as they get. One problem for girls – if the abuse comes from boys – is that there are no equivalent forms of speech for girls to use against boys. As Trudy told me:

One thing I noticed is that there are not many names you can call a boy. But if you call a girl a name, there's loads of them ... You might make a dictionary out of the names you can call a girl.

This lack of symmetry between the variety of names to call a girl and the lack of names to call boys is the starting point for an understanding of the role of verbal abuse which focuses on sexuality in reproducing, among girls, an orientation towards the existing structures of sex–gender relationships. The word which illustrates this asymmetry more clearly than any other term is 'slag'. There is no equivalent to 'slag' in the vocabulary of terms available to be directed at boys. Derogatory words for boys such as 'prick' or 'wally' are much milder in that they do not refer to the boys' social identity. 'Wally' is a word that can be used for both girls and boys to denote mild stupidity. To call a boy a 'poof' is derogatory but, according to girls, this term is not often used as a term of abuse by girls of boys. As a term used between boys, it implies lack of guts or femininity; which of itself connotes, in our culture, weakness, softness and inferiority. There is no derogatory word for active male sexuality. The promiscuous Don Juan or the stud may be rebuffed, as in Mozart's opera, but his reputation is enhanced. Sibyll describes how there is no vocabulary of abuse for girls to use and when asked how a girl can offend a boy replies:

Dunno. You can't say anything ... Perhaps if they go round with the girls all the time, they get called queers 'cos they're always with the girls ... You get some boys who like being in girls' company in a class, sitting with girls on the table.

If boys are seen as 'feminine' or are friendly with girls this can open them up to abuse. A young teacher described how in a single-sex boys' school a group of 'not real boys' or 'pseudo-girls' was constructed to delineate the borders between what was male and what was female: 'They are called the poofters and cissies and are constantly likened to girls. The sexual hierarchy gets set up but some boys have to play the part the girls would take in a mixed school' (Spender 1982).

The potency of 'slag' lies in the wide range of circumstances in which it can be used. It is this characteristic that illustrates its functioning as a form of generalized social control, along the lines of gender rather than class, steering girls, in terms of both their actions and their aspirations, into the existing structures of gender relations.

An alternative to asking those who use a term to define it is to observe carefully the rules whereby the term is used. A look at the actual usage of 'slag' reveals a wide variety of situations or aspects of behaviour to which the term can be applied, many of which are not related to a girl's actual sexual behaviour or to any clearly defined notion of 'sleeping around'. A constant sliding occurs between slag as a term of joking, as bitchy abuse, as a threat and as a label. What is more, and what makes it unique as a deviant category, is that it is never accepted by the recipients as applying to them. Drug addicts, for example, do not always deny their depiction. Alcoholics Anonymous see recognition of the label as the very first step to recovery. Yet no girl, however promiscuous, would admit to being a slag. This is borne out by Smith's study (1978) of delinquent girls, who are the ones typically ostracized as slags; they too reject the label and react aggressively against the accusation of 'easiness' contained in it. The label is shifted elsewhere, often to a group of girls who are in class terms 'inferior'. In other words, the shift is invariably socially downwards. What sense can be made of such labelling if the category is constantly being shifted across a wide range of girls amongst whom it is always another who embodies the term? It strikes me that it is the presence of the category which is important, not the identification of certain girls. Indeed, the notion of a small core of promiscuous girls, evidenced by the apparent fact that boys have more sexual partners than girls, remains more an assumption than an established fact. For the purpose of this analysis it becomes irrelevant to look for actual girls. Instead it seems more important to explore how the term is used. The following quotes should indicate some of the complexity of the term:

> At least the girls we go with ain't secondhand. (Conversation between boys baiting another boy – overheard by two girls in this study.)

At one moment a girl can be fanciable and the next 'a bit of a slag' or even – the other side of the coin – written off as 'too tight'. This is how a group of girls described what happens:

> BARBARA What I hate is when a boy tries, you go somewhere and a boy tries to sort of get in with you and if you dislike him as a person, then they say 'slag'. That's what really annoys me.
>
> Q *They'll say 'slag' if you don't want to go . . .*
> [*Interrupted by a chorus of 'Yeah, Yeah'.*]
>
> PAT 'Tight bitch', 'You tight bitch'. That sort of word.
>
> LINDA That's a terrible thing to say to someone – 'You're too tight.'
>
> PAT It's a vicious circle. If you don't like them, then they'll call you a tight bitch. If you go with them they'll call you a slag afterwards.

Girls must not end by being called a slag. But equally they do not want to be thought unapproachable, sexually cold – a tight bitch. Some boys took a fairly sophisticated view of how 'slag' was used:

> Q *What is a slag?*
>
> JOHN A girl who sleeps with loads of men or loads of boys.
>
> TOM Yeah.
>
> Q *At fifteen in your class?*
>
> JOHN In my class, I don't think so, no.
>
> Q *Yet girls are called slags?*
>
> JOHN Yeah. They use it as a nasty thing to say but with the meaning behind it. They mean it, yet they don't actually mean that the person sleeps with a load of boys all the time. They use it as a bad term.
>
> Q *What is the difference when girls use it?*

TOM They sort of use it like they would say 'you cow', or
something like that. It's different when girls use it.

Q *How is it different?*

TOM A girl doesn't feel so hurt when she's called it by a
girl. With a boy generally she'll just hit him. Chase him
around and beat him up. She might call him names.

Q *What names might she call him?*

TOM A poof or something like that.

Q *Why would she call him that?*

TOM To insult him. If a boy he's really macho then a
girl tells him he looks like a poof, he's not gonna like it.

Q *What does a poof look like?*

TOM Say he looks very feminine.

Earlier I commented that girls did not often call boys
'poofs' except in this situation where she is trying to bring a
'macho' boy down a peg or two. 'Poof' according to girls is
not a label they give to boys who are not macho.

The Ways in Which 'Slag' Can be Used

This constant sliding means that any girl is always available
for the designation 'slag', in any number of ways. Appearance
is crucial: by wearing too much make-up; by having your skirt
slit too high; by not combing your hair; by wearing jeans to
dances or high heels to school; by having your trousers too
tight or your tops too low. Trudy referred to these as 'sexual
clothes', implying that clothes are always seen in a sexual
context. Is it any wonder when girls have to learn to make
such fine distinctions about appearances that they spend so
much time deciding what to wear? Learning to be a girl
involves learning to sit with your legs together, learning not to
take up space and learning to dress appropriately. Tania,
working-class and black, describes how boys look at girls:

They look at people, like the trendy lot, and they think
that one's been fucked and that one's been fucked, but
they don't know, do they? They just say it 'cos they
wanna. She doesn't necessarily have had to be, does she?

Some clothes, however, indicate a lack of sexiness that can lead to a girl being classed as unattractive, 'a dog':

> The girl with the bell-bottoms and the beetle-crushers, she doesn't get called a slag. She doesn't get called nothing 'cos no one thinks – 'cos of her clothes – no one thinks that someone's had her.

This illustrates a crucial facet of 'slag', which is that it is both a despicable person but also an object of desire. She is sexy, as Sophie, middle-class and white, explains:

> I gotta think about that. She'll always wear tight trousers – a flirt – she'll have tight things on, or short things – sexual clothes. She'll have a lot of make-up on as well.

Sadie, a middle-class white girl, describes how being pretty can make a girl vulnerable, as it implies that she is sexually attractive. The girl who is unattractive would not be called a slag:

> Like Emma, this girl I know – that girl's been beat up so many times over things she's never done, y'know, like, she's been accused by some girls of going with one of the boys they fancy, when he's nothing to do with them. It's up to her, isn't it, and it's up to him, it's his preference. And they'll all jump on her when she's on her own, and there's about six of them. It's happened to her loads of times, it has. Maybe because she's pretty, that's why it could be, people just get jealous and that . . . accused her of being a slag when she's not.

The attractiveness of a girl is altered by having a reputation for easiness. Overt female sexuality has to be controlled:

> If you're a group of people, people get a reputation – she might be quite attractive, but where a slag can be unattractive is when she gets a reputation, so if a boy wants to sleep with someone, right, he'll say, 'Well, go and ask Maisie, you've got a chance there.' That's where it starts getting really awful – when you get a reputation.

Whom you mix with also counts:

> I prefer to hang around with someone who's a bit

decent, 'cos, I mean, if you walk down the street with someone who dresses weird you get a bad reputation yourself. Also if you look a right state, you'd get a bad reputation. 'Look at her,' y'know.

Looking weird often means dressing differently from your own group.

Behaviour towards boys is, of course, the riskiest terrain. The rules are strict. You must not hang around waiting for boys to come out too much (but all girls must hang around sufficiently); you must not talk or be friendly with too many boys or too many boys too quickly, or even more than one boy in a group; you must not find yourself ditched.

Almost everything plays a part in the constant assessment of reputation, including the way you speak:

> If we got a loud mouth, when we do the same [the boys] do, they call us slag, or 'got a mouth like the Blackwall tunnel'. But the boys don't get called that, when they go and talk. They think they're cool and hard and all the rest of it 'cos they can slag a teacher off.
>
> Q *Who would be calling you a slag then?*
>
> The boys they think, oh you got a mouth like an oar, you're all right down the fish market . . . They think you've come from a slum sort of area . . .

Thus 'slag' can just as easily be applied to a girl who dresses or talks in a certain way, or is seen talking to two boys or is seen with someone else's boyfriend. The point is that irrespective of whether in a particular case the use of the term 'slag' is applied explicitly to sexual behaviour, since a girl's reputation is defined in terms of her sexuality, all kinds of social behaviour by girls have a potent sexual significance.

There is nothing romantic in the girls' stark, indeed grim, appreciation of the state of gender relations and it is here that the term 'slag' is always pivoted. As Marina says:

> As soon as he's got it he'll drop you, and if you take too long to give it then he drops you anyway.
>
> Q *What do you think about sex?*

Oh I agree with it if you want it – I dunno. I'd hate to be pestered into it.

Q *How do you think boys are about it?*

I dunno. The girls always got fears about the boys going behind their backs and saying, 'Oh you know, had it with her' – they've always got that sort of thing.

Q *What's that fear about?*

I dunno, being called an old dog or something.

Q *By other girls or everybody?*

Everyone, but the girls are just as bad. You say to someone, 'How far did you get?' And she'll tell you and then you can always go to someone else and say, 'Oh she did, you know.'

The key to an understanding of 'slag' is its functioning as a mechanism that controls the activity and social reputations of girls to the advantage of boys. Girls were preoccupied with what might happen after being dropped by a boy:

Then the next thing he'll be going around saying, 'I've had her, you want to try her, go and ask her out. She's bound to say "Yeah".'

Or Shirley said:

Some boys are like that, they go round saying: 'I've had her,' and then they pack you in and their mate will go out with you. And you're thinking that they're going out with you 'cos they like you. But they're not. They're going out to use you. The next you know you're being called names – like writing on the wall: 'I've had it with so and so. I did her in three days. And I've done her twelve times in a week.'

It may not be a question of the girl actually having slept with a boy. She may land herself with a reputation as a result of going out with one boy, then being dropped and going out with one of his friends. The consequences for a girl are quite different from those for a boy:

When they're boys talking and you've been out with more than two you're known as the crisp that they're passing around ... The boy's all right but the girl's a bit of scum.

For some girls – especially girls who lead very restricted lives and are rarely allowed to go out (many from Bangladeshi and Greek families for example) – even being known to frequent certain places is enough to risk your reputation. A Greek girl, Rona, whose father works in a restaurant, describes this process:

> If at the age of fourteen she starts going out, they say that no boy will want to marry her when she's older if they find out she's been going out. I know a lot of boys who would say 'I wouldn't go out with a girl that's been to so-and-so places.' Just because she's been to that place, it doesn't mean she's bad. But you get a bad reputation because of the place – like some way-out discos. I know a boy, he goes, 'If I found out that my fiancée went out to that disco, I'd leave her straight-away,' he goes. Not that she did anything. It's just that, y'know, the place gives you a bad name even if you've only been once.

It is not only boys who call girls slags. Girls are constantly accusing girls of being slags, usually when they are jealous. Jealousy can arise from the way a girl dresses or if she is found talking to someone else's boyfriend or if she is pretty:

> Tracy's called names because they think she's too trendy. We went to this careers conference and there were loads of other schools there and we were the only sort of trendy school there. Insults were hurled at all of us, especially Tracy. It was horrible. I thought they shouldn't be like that when they don't even know her. Just because of her clothes ... It gets me when people say, 'Oh, she's a slag. She does this and she does that.' But a lot of it is jealousy, 'cos they don't do it themselves. They're jealous that she's got more than them.

Particular risks are run in relation to a girl's reputation if birth-control and contraceptives are used. If a girl takes contraceptives on a casual date this involves laying herself open to

savage criticism, because it is premeditated sex, which contravenes the 'dominant code of romance'. On the other hand to
have sex without contraceptives is even more risky, particularly
now with the risk of AIDS, which will be discussed in detail
in Chapter 5. As one girl explains, to become pregnant on a
casual date proves to others that you must be a slag:

> If she got pregnant then everyone thinks, 'Oh my God,
> she really has been sleeping with him,' like where you
> can't really imagine it. If she's pregnant you know she
> has – you literally know it and then they say 'Oh God,
> she's so cheap . . .' Then it'll just go round.

The main risk then is that the boy will turn out to be a
'boaster' and will spread stories about you after he has chucked
you. It is therefore unwise to sleep with a boy too quickly in
case, as a number of girls said, 'he is using you' and will be off
the moment he has got what he wants. Even if you have known
a boy some time it is impossible to be sure that he will not go
round spreading tales about you. As Marianne, working-class,
living with three brothers, comments in a group discussion:

> He could have been good all the way until you went to
> bed with him. Then as soon as he'd got that from you,
> he's off, just saying, 'had my piece from her. It's all right
> now,' and off he goes and news travels around.

Girls agreed that there were some boys who boast about it
and others who don't. Debbie knows some boys are to be avoided:

> One who thinks he's a Casanova, thinks he can have
> every bird. I know a lot of people like that. They're
> there rabbiting away to you about – saying I think
> you're beautiful all that stuff – and they think you're
> taking it in but you're just sitting there ignoring it
> because they think they're Casanovas.

All the girls agreed that when it comes down to it you can't
be sure which kind of boy you're dealing with. Boys behave
very differently when they are with their friends. After interviewing girls from two schools with a predominantly working-
class intake, we repeated the study in a single-sex school with

a high middle-class intake. Though there were some differences in the way girls handled abuse, few differences were found in the way girls described their relations with boys and the way they categorized other girls in terms of their sexual reputation, and indeed were categorized themselves. Some of the black girls appeared more confident and aware of sexism than the white girls.

In reviewing her study of fourteen-year-old girls, Angela McRobbie found that there was a disparity between her 'wheeling in' of class in her report and its complete absence from the girls' talk and discourse. She concluded that being working-class meant little or nothing to these girls, but being a girl over-determined their every moment (McRobbie 1982). Girls are aware of class differences in income, accent, access to a wider social life and better opportunities, but the objectification of girls occurs regardless of class, though middle-class girls may have access to greater linguistic practices to deal with abuse. However, any girl or woman can be brought down to size by being rendered a bitch, a cow or a cunt, which girls regard as deeply offensive, but is also one of the few words to describe the female sex organs. One distinction that did emerge in the discussions with middle-class girls was a greater awareness that the defining characteristic of 'slag' was not in fact actual promiscuity. As Silvia, a middle-class white girl from a single-sex school, explains:

> There are some people I know who have slept with lots of different people, but they don't conduct themselves in a way that I would call a slag, they don't do it on purpose, they don't sort of treat boys in a completely different way – grease up to them and change their whole personality because someone they like is in the room kind of thing, and some people who have slept with different people I wouldn't define as a slag.
>
> Q *Why would you have defined the two girls as slags?*
>
> Because they were using people and became very flirtatious. You wouldn't recognize them as the same people. You

could be having a conversation with them one minute. Someone they like comes into the room, suddenly they change their whole personalities. They don't talk to you sincerely. It's tits out. And then all they want of the boys is to get off with them. They'd go off with two, three boys.

Q *Do you mean they'd be sleeping with three people?*

Oh no, I didn't mean they'd be sleeping, but, I mean, that would be a bit hard.

The girl here is describing behaviour that would be regarded as natural in a boy. It is natural for a boy to chat up girls. Here if a girl is seen to be appearing to chat up boys or perhaps talking to three different boys in succession she is in danger of being regarded as a slag. What Silvia fails to appreciate is the constraints on a girl, the limits on her freedom to move around, to talk to whoever she wants and behave independently. Such behaviour would be categorized as inappropriately forward, attention-seeking and 'sluttish'. There are ways in which stereotypes of class, such as low intelligence and rough language, overlap with sexist abuse. In the same way that 'slut' denotes both promiscuity and low social class, Anna Marie describes Tania, whom she regards as stupid, in this way:

This girl I know – she couldn't even pass her entrance into Woolworths. And usually they come from very poor families. I never ask them to go out with us.

Peter Wilmott, in his study of boys, found a connection between swearing and assumed looseness. He quotes one of the boys he interviewed as saying: 'You can always get a bit with the girls with big mouths, but that kind of thing turns you off after a while – you realize that if you can get it so can anyone else' (Wilmott 1969).

The Effect of Sexist Abuse

The crucial point about the label 'slag' is that it is used by both girls and boys as a deterrent to nonconformity. No girl wants to be labelled 'bad', and 'slag' is something to frighten any girl with. As Laura said, 'Everyone thinks lower of them than what they did before.' The effect of the term is to force girls to submit voluntarily to a very unfair set of gender relations. A few girls did reject the implications of the label and the double standard implicit within it, but even they said they used the term to abuse other girls.

To call a girl a slag is to use a term that, as we have seen, appears at first sight to be a label describing an actual form of behaviour but into which no girl incontrovertibly fits. It is even difficult to identify what actual behaviour is specified. Take Helen's description of how appearance can define girls, not in terms of their attributes as human beings, but in terms of sexual reputation:

> I mean, they might not mean any harm. I mean, they might not be as bad as they look. But their appearance makes them stand out and that's what makes them look weird and you think: 'God, I can imagine her, y'know?' . . . She straight away gets a bad reputation even though the girl might be decent inside. She might be good. She might still be living at home. She might just want to look different but might still act normal.

You cannot imagine a boy's appearance being described in this way. How she dresses determines how a girl is viewed and she is viewed in terms of her assumed sexual behaviour. Whether she is 'good' or not is determined by how she is assumed to conduct her sexual life; that sexuality is relative to male sexual needs. Girls are aware that appearances may be deceptive, but this does not lead them to really contest the categorization:

> You can't tell a slag walking down the street. I mean, you might see someone who looks a real – debauched, sort of mess, make-up run everywhere, but you don't know the reason. You might call her a slag, but, I mean, she could just have been beaten up by her husband or something. So really a slag is usually someone you know and you just have evidence of what they've done.

Rather than attempt to specify what particular behaviour

differentiates a slag, it is more useful to see 'slag' as what Sumner (1983) terms a category of 'moral censure': as part of a discourse about male conceptions of female sexuality that run deep in the culture. They run so deep that the majority of women and men cannot formulate them except by reference to these terms of censure that signal a threatened violation.

Their general function is to denounce and control, not to explain . . . They mark off the deviant, the pathological, the dangerous and the criminal from the normal and the good . . . [they] are not just labels . . . [But] . . . They are loaded with implied interpretations of real phenomena, models of human nature and the weight of political self interest (Sumner 1983).

What Sumner fails to explore is how these forms of moral censure are gendered. In effect exactly the behaviour which would be extolled in a boy is censured in a girl. 'Slag' is literally the coal dust that is 'cast off' on to the slag heap, or, in sexual terms, the woman who is fucked and discarded. However, it is also one of the few words to imply active female sexuality, personified in the prostitute. The term is of course highly derogatory, yet it refers to a woman who behaves in the way men are expected to behave. A slag is a woman who is 'after one thing', someone 'who does not really care', or 'uses sex for other motives' rather than love (the whore who has sex for money). For a man to have sex without a relationship is fine, to be expected, part of 'natural male sex drive'. In one discussion with adolescent boys, Nico, hearing I had had discussions with girls, was curious as to what they had said about sex. 'Do girls like sex?' he asked as though the question had never crossed his mind before.

We shall see in Chapter 7 what strategies girls adopt to deal with abuse, how they often react by denying the accusations rather than by objecting to the use of the category. It is important to prove that you are not a slag. So Wendy, when asked what she'd do if someone called her a slag, replied, 'I'd turn round and say "Why? Tell me why?"'

For girls to have sex for its own sake makes them into 'prostitutes'. It could be argued that both prostitutes and men separate their bodies from their emotions: the prostitute has sex for money, the man for conquest. So for a girl sex is only legitimate when she interacts with the boy, when she 'recognizes' the boy, when she likes him, not when she treats the boy as an object of her desire. To demand sex for itself makes her dirty, destroys her 'womanliness'. This is relevant to the construction of female sexuality. The loss of virginity represents a cheapening of the woman, a drop in her value. Amazingly, in the interviews I undertook with boys, many of whom were actively having sex with girls, they still voiced a commitment to finding a virgin to marry. In some cultures a loss of virginity precludes the possibility of marriage. Paul Willis suggests that there is a fear that unleashing the woman's desire will lead to uncontrolled promiscuity. In analysing the term 'slag' as a representation he comments: 'Woman . . . as a sexual object is a commodity that becomes worthless with consumption and yet as a sexual being, once sexually experienced, becomes promiscuous.' He quotes one of his lads as saying: 'After you've been with one, like, after you've done it, like, well, they're scrubbers afterwards, they'll go with anyone. I think that once they've had it, they want it all the time, no matter who it's with' (Willis 1977).

The term slag therefore applies less to any clearly defined notion of sleeping around than to any form of social behaviour by girls that would define them as autonomous from the attachment to and domination by boys. It acts as a censure against being unattached. In other words, any independent behaviour – such as going places on your own, or talking back to a boy, or standing your ground in a dispute – opens a girl up to sexist abuse. A second important facet of 'slag' is its uncontested status as a category. Although it connotes promiscuity, its actual usage is such that any unattached girl is vulnerable to being categorized as a slag. In this way the term functions as a form of control by boys over girls, a form of control that steers girls into 'acceptable' and dependent forms

of sexual and social behaviour. The term is uncontestable. All
the girls agreed that there was only one defence, one way for a
girl to redeem herself from the reputation of slag:

> To get a steady boyfriend. Then that way you seem to
> be more respectable, like you're married or something.

'Going steady' establishes the location of a sexuality appropriate for 'nice girls', and that sexuality is distinguished from
the essentially dirty/promiscuous sexuality of the slag. Sex
with a steady boyfriend is easy to get away with:

> If you had it away with your boyfriend, right, and you
> didn't tell no one, no one else needs to know, do they?

It is the young unattached woman who is likely to be
regarded as a slag, rather than the sexually active girl who
sleeps with her boyfriend. The term slag functions as a pressure
on girls to submit to a relationship of dependence on a boy,
leading eventually to marriage. It is this complex nexus of
constraints that lies behind the importance all girls lay on
finding a boyfriend and leads to girls often colluding in their
own oppression. Being unattached carries risks:

> If you went round with someone, right, or you don't know
> her but you always see her and every time you see her
> she's got a different fella with her, you get to think she's
> a slag, don't you? She got a different fella every minute
> of the day.

The following interview with Jacky illustrates the way the
slag categorization shifts away from girls who have settled
down with a boyfriend on to the girl who is still unattached:

> I don't call a slag someone who just happens to, like,
> who desperately wants a boyfriend, so they'll get a boy-
> friend, then he chucks her a week later, so she gets
> another one, so like over a period of three months she
> might have been seen with six boys.
> Q *So she'll get called a slag just because she's been seen with six
> different boys?*
> If you see them with a different person. This friend of
> ours, Brenda, like she – everyone I know, like Helen and

Sally – they call her a slag. I often get so angry with them
'cos I think she's just unlucky, she just happens to go around
with a group of people. She went out with one, then he
chucked her, then with the other one, another boy, so she
went out with him and she genuinely likes him. She
genuinely wants to go with him. She just happens to be
unlucky enough to be dropped by them all and they're sort
of saying, 'Oh, who is she with tonight?'

Q *Why do they call her a slag?*

It's hypocritical, though, because I would define them as
slags at one point.

Q *Why would you define them as slags?*

At one time, not at the moment, but because they've
settled now with a steady boyfriend, or whatever. They
think that other people are doing what they're doing.
It's wrong. There was a time when they just went to a
party, they'd go off with some boy like and an hour later
they'd go off with another. That is what I consider a
slag. It's completely debauched, sort of not really caring.

As we have seen, calling a girl a slag can have nothing to do
with sex but can just be directed at a girl who flirts or is seen
with a number of different boys. The reason why they are
defined or labelled as slags is, as Jacky implies, that they are
unattached. Helen and Sally are no longer seen as slags as
they have settled with steady boyfriends, yet this does not
stop them branding Brenda as a slag when she is unattached.
Jacky objects to this on the grounds that it is unfair: Brenda
does not fall into her concept of what a slag is. Once she is
labelled a slag the language of the consumer society emerges.
It cheapens a girl if she sleeps with a boy. Here we can see not
only how women's bodies are seen as commodities, but also
that the value of them depends not simply on their attractiveness but on the girls' reputations as well.

Any girl is always available to the designation 'slag' in any
number of ways, as we have seen. It is clearly a very narrow
tightrope to walk to achieve sexual attractiveness without the
taint of sexuality. How the criteria for such discrimination are

generated remains obscure. What is certain is that the criteria shift from group to group, from individual to individual. The boys are not clear to whom the term refers, as two researchers found when interviewing boys in a London housing estate:

The boys classified all the girls into two categories: the slags who'd go with anyone and everyone (they were all right for a quick screw, but you'd never get serious about it) and the drags who didn't but who you might one day think about going steady with. Different cliques of boys put different girls in each of the two categories (Robbins and Cohen 1978:58).

Despite the apparent connection between the designation 'slag' and sexual promiscuity, the term has probably very little to do with actual sexual behaviour, as the following quote perhaps more than any other indicates:

MANDY Like this girl that I know, this boy that she used to go out with, right, he started calling her names, and so all his friends started calling her names.

Q *What sort of names?*

MANDY Like slag, prostitute, whore, all those things.

Q *While she was going out with him?*

MANDY No, after she had finished with him. He went round saying that she couldn't kiss, see, 'cos she sort of gets embarrassed, she's like that over the slightest thing. He stayed with her for four months and then he goes round saying she couldn't kiss. I admit she only kissed him once, but he knows that is why she wouldn't because she was embarrassed and that and he went round saying that she couldn't kiss and yet he's saying she's a slag and all. So I thought to myself, how could he stay with her for four months and go round saying that? He really liked her, he would have bought her anything. It's too bad.

The boy here is calling his girlfriend, who is too shy and embarrassed to kiss, a slag. The lack of connection between sexual promiscuity and sexual abuse could hardly be greater.

Concern about teenage pregnancy centring mainly on the

independence of teenage mothers is a frequent theme in the media. Teenage girls are seen both as powerfully seductive and as 'easy to get'. As Sharon and Marion describe it:

MARION 'Cos I think many girls, once you're sixteen, eighteen, they think you're easy to get.

SHARON Yes. The girls put on a lot of make-up and they go into the pub or something, y'know, nudge, nudge. She's all right, force her to have sex and afterwards when she's pregnant abandon her and leave her alone. It's just like that.

MARION Yeah, a toy.

SHARON Play with it and then chuck it away like it's broken.

This reputation for easiness can lead to a girl being beaten up by girls. It is often the girls who mete out retribution on a girl who is known to contravene the dominant code of sexual conduct. Laura describes the kind of episode that can occur:

My friend knows this girl and she's a bit of a tart and she invites boys to her house and once these skinheads came along and she started taking her clothes off and everything and these boys said they didn't have any girlfriends but the girls were waiting outside and they brought their girlfriends in and beat her up and everything and she was in hospital, so now no one takes any notice of her or anything, they just leave her to herself.

Q *The girls beat her up?*

Yes, the boys as well, kicked her about and everything.

Q *What do you think about that?*

It was her own fault, she shouldn't do it – it's horrible. Mind you, two wrongs don't make a right.

What is of particular interest here is the operation of an ideology that transforms the experience of very unfair relations between the sexes into an acceptance of those relations as natural. It is somehow wrong and horrible for a girl to invite sexual activity, but somehow natural for the boy to be after it, to attempt to pester you into it, to tell if you do and to fabricate its occurrence if you don't. If a girl contravenes this code she deserves to be beaten up. Fear of getting a bad reputation stopped some girls from going out:

> It makes you feel terrible, makes you feel as if you don't wanna go out. Say soon as you go outside the door you get someone calling you a slag. It's not worth it.

Evidence from research carried out in other countries suggests that a girl's reputation is analysed in a similar way, though the vocabulary of abuse may differ. In *Louts and Legends*, for example, an Australian study of teenage boys, Walker describes how

Girls' behaviour and reputations were analysed using a range of categories from 'maddie', 'nympho' and 'mole' to 'stiff' and 'darling'. Maddies or nymphos were believed to have insatiable sexual appetites, and might also be moles if they were thought indiscriminating about partners, were easily pushed around, or were dressed (in very tight clothes) or moved (e.g. suggestively elbowing boys in the ribs) in a manner perceived as crudely provocative. Stiffs (males can also be stiffs) are perceived as physically strong and sexually attractive, darlings stimulate romantic yearnings (Walker 1988:108).

Racist and Sexist Stereotyping

In the same way that girls are aware of class differences, they are also aware of ethnic differences. Black girls are not a homogeneous group, and very different types of gender relations exist among different groups.

The relation between cultural backgrounds has already been mentioned in relation to the importance of *izzat* or family honour in some Asian households. Religious customs and beliefs operate in such a way as to control female sexuality in so far as most religions lay down moral codes relating to virginity and sexual behaviour. One of the main ethnic differences that emerged was the amount of freedom girls are allowed, to go out late, or at all, and to mix with boys of religions different to those of their own families. Some girls' lives are much more constricted than others, which is as much related to their families' religious beliefs as to race. Work is also liberating many women from total dependence. In the case of Asian women during the last ten years, going out to work, if only part-time, is breaking the knot of total dependence some experienced (see Westwood and Bhachu 1988).

There is a sense in which racist and sexist stereotyping are intertwined and related. The sexist category of 'slag' is part of the raw material out of which racist views are elaborated. Sexist and racist stereotypes operate in ways which, although not identical, are in some respects similar. Both sets of stereotypes are difficult to pin down to any hard or specific content that could be shown to be untrue and thus lead to the withdrawal of the label. For 'slag' this is because of the ambiguous way in which it is used; in the case of racist stereotypes this results from a refusal to allow any exceptions. Gordon Allport (1954), an American social psychologist who, after the Second World War, carried out a classic study of prejudice to try and throw light on the horrors of the Holocaust, called this re-fencing.

There is a common mental device that permits people to hold to prejudgements even in the face of much contradictory evidence. It is the device of admitting exceptions. 'There are nice Negroes but . . .' Or, 'Some of my best friends are Jews but . . .' This is a disarming device. By excluding a few favoured cases, the negative rubric is kept intact for all other cases. In short, contrary evidence is not admitted and allowed to modify the generalization; rather it is perfunctorily acknowledged but excluded (Allport 1954:23).

This process of acknowledging and then excluding exceptions is illustrated by a snippet of conversation where Karen elaborates on the sexual and racial prejudices of herself and her friends:

Like me . . . Pam and me and Susan . . . and we were sat in those flats talking, and I just said . . . A Paki come along, and Pam says, 'Oh, I hate Pakis,' and I go, 'Oh, I hate Jews,' and Susan goes, 'I hate black people.' And I go, 'How can you hate black people? Sybil's black,' and, like, Susan and Pamela and me were all white, and she goes, 'I don't really' . . . She goes, 'I hate golliwogs.' 'My best friend's black,' and she goes, 'Yeah, so's mine,' so I go 'Yeah? So

how can you hate them?' and Pamela goes, 'I hate Pakis.'
. . . No reason, she just hates them. I hate Jews for a reason.

Karen's reason for hating Jews is that:

A Jew knocked my dog down and he died, so ever since
then I've hated Jews and I hate all Jews.

Q *You think all Jews are like that?*

Yeah now. Only them that wear the black thing and . . . I
had a Jewish friend and I didn't know she was Jewish and
I was watching *Jesus of Nazareth* up her house one day
and I said to her when the Jews come on, I said, 'Oh,
look, the Jews,' and she said, 'I'm Jewish,' and her dad
was there and all and she goes her dad's Jewish – he's
not one of them Jews that wear the black thing . . . Ever
since then I don't play with her.

Q *Do you like her?*

No not a lot. That weren't the only reason I didn't like
her. There were other reasons but that made it worse.

Karen's incoherence illustrates both sides of the process that
Allport was describing. On the one hand, a counterfactual
example to a racist generalization will happily be incorporated
without disturbing the generalization, and on the other hand, a
single instance will be held up as sufficient reason for subscribing
to a generalization about an ethnic or religious group.

Thus both the 'slag' and racist categorizations are forms of
labelling that are difficult to pin down to any specific content
that could be shown to be untrue and lead to a withdrawal of
the label. For 'slag', this is because of the ambiguous way in
which it is used. In the case of race it is by refusing to allow
any exception to modify the basic racist stereotype. It is easy
to see how 'slag' can come to fulfil the requirements of racism.
Racist stereotypes of blacks and whites occur among the girls
through the familiar devices of 'slag' and bitching, which are
at the same time being used by both girls and boys in ways
that end up constraining the freedom of girls, irrespective of
ethnic group. The processes by which girls are labelled 'slags',
irrespective of race, can become one component out of which
racist views are elaborated. It is not just that 'slag' is a label

that has a fluidity similar to racist stereotypes. Racism is able to absorb and work through sexist categories. In *Black Women in White America* Gerda Lerner explains the centrality of sexual mythology concerning black women:

By assuming a different level of sexuality for all blacks than that of whites and mystifying their greater sexual potency, the black woman could be made to personify sexual freedom and abandon. A myth was created that all black women were eager for sexual exploits, voluntarily 'loose' in their morals, and therefore deserved none of the consideration and respect granted white women. Every black woman was, by definition, a slut according to racist mythology; therefore to assault her and exploit her sexually was not reprehensible and carried with it none of the normal sanctions against such behaviour (Lerner 1981, quoted in hooks 1981:59).

This 'animal' sexual appetite and behaviour of the black woman finds a reflection in a comment by a white girl in this study:

> They look black and somehow stronger. If you got a white girl and a black girl you say, 'Oh she looks stronger 'cos she's black.'

Appearance is important in the process of racial as well as sexual stereotyping. The awareness of dress differences is a key theme in the feelings of racial antagonism between black and white girls in the public spaces outside the classroom. Jane, a white girl, describes how it is the black girls she is most frightened of when she goes out, and that if you dress like some black girls – wearing brightly coloured cotton – then you are 'asking for it':

> Then we went to the Lyceum, all of us looked really smart, and there was this group of black girls and they were all going 'Tchch' and looking us up and down, and you feel uneasy with them.

Black girls feel themselves on the receiving end of innuendo concerning dress from white girls. Wilma complains about the way

> They tease you about the way you dress, sometimes the way you walk . . . [The white girls] think they're perfect, that's why. They say something to you and when you say it back

they say, 'What did you say it about me for?' They don't like it. They can say it to you but you can't say it to them.

This is echoed by Sharon:

Some of [the white girls] are all trendy, the sort of dresses and that, and then there're some of them that are really bitchy. The thing that gets me is they take the piss out of our clothes and then half of their clothes come from jumble sales. I couldn't get my clothes from a jumble sale.

This bitching about clothes is of course no different from relations between girls in terms of subcultural styles. A white girl talks about trendies in much the same way:

They might not mean any harm, they might not be that bad, as bad as they look, but their appearance makes them stand out and that's what makes them look weird and you think, 'God, I can imagine her'. . . Straight away she gets a bad reputation even though she might be decent inside.

What this illustrates is not that racism is 'just another' form of bitching between girls over dress and style of behaviour, but rather that racism constructs its stereotypes out of the content of everyday interpersonal interaction which is then institutionalized (otherwise racism appears as only interactive). The processes by which girls are labelled slags, irrespective of race, are one component of the way in which racial stereotypes are constructed and perpetuated. Black women are therefore seen by these girls to be particularly sexy. As Lynne Segal (1987:102) indicates, western images of sex are also quintessentially racist.

We have seen that the vocabulary used to describe girls divides them into good and bad, the promiscuous and the pure, the tasty and the 'dogs'. It is not only the boys that categorize girls in this way but girls use the same terms to categorize and 'police' each other. Embodied in this vocabulary is a contempt for women which emerges if they are seen to be actively sexual and unattached. What is particularly pernicious about this language is that it is accepted as part of nature, or of common sense, by the girls themselves.

Sometimes other members of the family are brought into arguments about a girl's reputation. Both fathers and brothers were reported to call girls slags, which gives the nasty impression that they might be involved in other forms of abuse, perhaps sexual abuse. Sadie said that when her dad called her a slag, her mum retorted:

> Look at your sister. She was pregnant at sixteen. So you can't talk about your daughter like that.

Sybil, when asked what she thought about her brothers, replied:

> I ain't got no brothers really. All they do is call me names, especially the eldest one. Then the other two join in.

Sexual abuse in childhood and adolescence can be a devastating experience for women in terms of their body image and overall self-esteem. American studies estimate that as many as one in three girls are sexually abused (Russell 1984). Alice Miller outlines the drastic effects if children are beaten, humiliated, lied to and deceived, and how anger, if unexpressed, does not disappear but is transformed with time into a more or less conscious hatred against either the self or a substitute person (Miller 1987).

Conclusions

An absence of any form of expression of sexual desire among girls except in terms of an exclusive 'love' relationship is one significant finding. Yet there is talk about who did what, with whom and how far they went. But all this talk is circumscribed and checked by the invocation of the category 'slag'. Far from being personal and private, sexuality reflects unfair power relations between the sexes. Girls are categorized as passive objects who can only wait and hope to be chatted up without being insulted, to make love and not be talked about afterwards. The terms on which their dilemmas are handled are always socially organized and largely socially determined. Girls may have more freedom, but they have to develop strategies for dealing with day-to-day sexism. Some are voicing their rejection of the double standard. There may be little collective protest but some girls are questioning sexism. Girls tease each other for playing up to boys. Girls are having fun, and can be humorous, self-assured and full of spark. Girls do not passively accept their subordination. Yet feminism is more popular among women who have had children than among adolescents, who are too preoccupied with developing ways of surviving the contradictions of female identity.[3]

In this chapter I have shown how femininity and masculinity are socially constituted and reconstituted through social practices and are not biologically determined. For the adolescent girls I spoke to feminine identity rests to a great extent on their sexual reputation. The only terms for active female sexuality are derogatory. Otherwise, girls are categorized as passive objects. The terms on which their dilemmas are handled are always socially organized and largely socially determined. Defining girls in terms of their sexual reputation rather than their attributes and potentialities is a crucial mechanism of ensuring their subordination to boys. The lack of specific content of the term 'slag' means that girls are in a permanent state of vulnerability, for the way they dress and speak, for being too friendly to boys or not friendly enough. The terms of abuse are so taken for granted that girls do not often question them; they use the terms of abuse themselves against other girls. The only security against abuse and a bad reputation is to confine themselves to the 'protection' of one partner. Yet such a resolution involves dependency and loss of autonomy, as I shall elaborate in Chapter 3.

Notes

1. See Sharpe 1976, Wilson 1978, Griffin 1985, Brumberg 1988, Holly 1989, Campbell 1981, 1984, Sharpe 1987, Stafford 1991, Walkerdine 1990, Weiner 1985, Gaskell 1992.
2. According to a study released in 1991 commissioned by the

American Association of University Women, only 29 per cent of
female students in high school said they were 'happy the way I am'
compared with 46 per cent of boys. Black women had higher self-
esteem but reported more feelings of alienation from school and
teachers than their white counterparts.

   3. Gloria Steinem (1979) found that older women become
more radical as a result of their experiences with men. Younger
women are more conservative.

Bibliography

Allport, G., 1954, *The Nature of Prejudice*, Addison Wesley
Amos, V., and Parmar, P., 1987, 'Resistances and Responses: The
    Experiences of Black Girls in Britain', in Arnot, M., and Weiner,
    G. (eds.), *Gender and the Politics of Schooling*, pp. 211–22, Oxford
    University Press
Arnot, M., 1982, 'How Shall We Educate Our Sons?', in Deems, R.
    (ed.), *Coeducation Reconsidered*, Open University Press
Black, M., and Coward, R., 1981, 'Linguistic, Social and Sexual
    Relations', in *Screen Education*, 39
Brah, A., and Minhas, R., 1985, 'Structural Racism and Cultural
    Difference: Schooling for Asian Girls', in Weiner, G., *Just a
    Bunch of Girls*, pp. 14–25, Open University Press
Brumberg, J., 1988, *Fasting Girls*, Harvard University Press
Campbell, A., 1981, *Girl Delinquents*, Blackwell
Campbell, A., 1984, *Girls in the Gang*, Blackwell
Connell, B., Radican, N., and Martin, P., 1987, *The Changing Faces of
    Masculinity*, Macquarie University
Davies, B., 1989, *Frogs and Snails and Feminist Tales*, Allen and Unwin
Gaskell, J., 1992, *Gender Matters: From School to Work*, Oxford Univer-
    sity Press
Griffin, C., 1985, *Typical Girls*, Routledge and Kegan, Paul
Hancock, E., 1990, *The Girl Within, A Radical New Approach to Female
    Identity*, Pandora
Holly, L., 1989, *Girls and Sexuality: Teaching and Learning*, Oxford
    University Press
hooks, b., 1981, *Ain't I a Woman*, South End Press
Lerner, G., 1981, *Black Women in White America*, quoted in bel hooks,
    1983, *Ain't I a Woman*

McRobbie, A., 1982, 'The Politics of Feminist Research: Between Talk, Text and Action', in *Feminist Review*, 12

Miller, A., 1987, *For Your Own Good: The Roots of Violence in Child-rearing*, Virago

Raymond, J., 1991, *A Passion for Friends*, Women's Press

Robbins, D., and Cohen, P., 1978, *Knuckle Sandwich*, Penguin

Russell, D., 1984, *Sexual Exploitation: Rape, Child Sexual Abuse and Workplace Harassment*, Sage

Segal, L., 1987, *Is the Future Female*, Virago

Sharpe, S., 1976, *Just Like a Girl*, Penguin

Sharpe, S., 1987, *Falling for Love*, Virago Upstarts

Spender, D., 1980, *Man Made Language*, Routledge and Kegan Paul

Spender, D., 1982, *Invisible Women*, Writers and Readers Press

Spender, D., and Sarah, E. (eds.), 1980, *Learning to Lose*, Women's Press

Stafford, A., 1991, *Trying Work*, Edinburgh University Press

Steinem, G., 1979, 'Why Young Women are More Conservative', in *Ms* magazine, reprinted in *Outrageous Acts and Everyday Rebellions*, 1986, Signet, pp. 238–46

Sumner, C., 1983, 'Rethinking Deviance Towards a Sociology of Censures', *Research in Law, Deviance and Social Control*, Vol. 5, JAI Press

Walker, J. C., 1988, *Louts and Legends: Male Youth Culture in an Inner-City School*, Allen and Unwin

Walkerdine, V., 1990, *Schoolgirl Fictions*, Verso

Weiner, G., 1985, *Just a Bunch of Girls*, Oxford University Press

Westwood, S., and Bhachu, P. (eds.), 1988, *Enterprising Women: Ethnicity, Economy and Gender Relations*, Routledge and Kegan Paul

Willis, P., 1977, *Learning to Labour*, Saxon House

Wilmott, P., 1969, *Adolescent Boys in East London*, Penguin

Wilson, A., 1978, *Finding a Voice*, Virago

Chapter 2
Friendship

From the days of Homer the friendships of men have enjoyed glory
and acclamation, but the friendships of women, in spite of Ruth and
Naomi, have usually been not merely unsung, but mocked, belittled
and falsely interpreted (Vera Brittain 1947)

The failure to examine heterosexuality as an institution is like failing
to admit that the economic system called capitalism or the caste
system of racism is maintained by a variety of forces, including both
physical violence and false consciousness (Rich 1980:648)

In what way are girls' friendships similar to boys' and in what
way are they different? In this chapter I illustrate the importance of friendship in girls' lives, and the growing recognition
that friendship is important for girls and women as well as for
men. I examine the mechanisms by which their relationships
are dominated by gender relations and how female friendship
can both protect and undermine a girl's sexual reputation. I
then consider how and why girls' friendships change when
they get a boyfriend and why they generally prioritize relationships with men.

In the extensive literature on the family, marriage and
motherhood, friendship is scarcely mentioned. Female friendship has received so little attention that some question whether
it exists or whether women have the capacity for it. Lionel
Tiger, an eminent social psychologist, unequivocally maintained that women lack the bonding instinct that binds men
together in groups (Tiger 1969). I remember arguing with my
father-in-law, a bus-driver for forty years, about whether
women had friends – in spite of the fact that his wife spent
many hours on the telephone to her friends and many evenings
meeting them. To acknowledge friendship among women is to

give them autonomy, an existence apart from men and male interests. Simone de Beauvoir pinpoints this when she says, 'If woman did not exist, man would have invented her. But she exists also apart from their inventiveness' (de Beauvoir 1972:174). If she exists in relation to other women, she is not confined to a male identified world. Women have been friends through the ages, but their friendships have been dismembered, not merely rendered invisible but denied on the grounds that women are too busy competing for men. In this tradition, Simone de Beauvoir depicts female friendship as 'Rarely rising to genuine friendship . . . as they all face together the masculine world, whose values they wish to monopolize each for herself . . . And so in the sphere of coquetry and love each woman sees in every other an enemy' (de Beauvoir 1972:558).

More positively, Virginia Woolf describes her surprise when she first read a novel written by a woman that portrayed female friendship. 'Chloe liked Olivia. Olivia liked Chloe for perhaps the first time in literature.' She goes on to speculate on what our past might have been like if relationships between women had ever been the focus: 'So often women are not seen by the other sex, but only in relation to the other sex. So common sense even dictates that women are not really capable of friendship – or at least real friendship' (Woolf 1929).

Friendship and Adolescent Girls

I mean a real friend is someone who's loyal and won't go around talking about you, and she'll stick up for you and she won't bitch about you. And when you are depressed or something you can just go and talk to her. To be on your side rather than on someone else's, even if they don't agree. They'll stick up for you and then afterwards they'll say I sticked up for you but I don't agree with you (Rosie, aged fifteen).

In the late 1970s Angela McRobbie, one of the few British

sociologists to undertake a study of girls and their friendships, argued that the absence of girls from studies of youth needed explaining; she pointed out that very little had been written about the role of girls in general: 'They are absent from the classical subcultural ethnographic studies; the pop histories, personal accounts or journalistic surveys' (McRobbie and Garber 1976).

She asked whether this was due to the dominance of male sociologists (many of whom she suggested had a particular fascination with the macho image of male subcultures), or whether to the specifically masculine nature of most subcultures. She concluded that girls were only marginally present in boys' groups and that their marginal presence was simply a reproduction of their 'cultural subordination'. She went on to inquire whether there were equivalent female youth collective experiences producing their own strategies; whether there were complementary ways in which girls interact among themselves and with each other to form a distinctive culture of their own:

When the dimension of sexuality is included in the study of subcultures, girls can be seen to be negotiating a different space, offering a different type of resistance to what can at least in part be viewed as their sexual subordination (McRobbie and Garber 1976:221).

The important question, according to McRobbie, is not the absence or presence of girls in the male subcultures, but whether they form distinctive cultures of their own ... 'The subcultural grouping may not be the most likely place where those equivalent rituals, responses and negotiations will be located.' Since at least at this age, girls are much more home based than boys, and spend much time with two or three friends listening to records and talking about boys and pop stars, she called this a 'bedroom culture'. This bedroom culture is described as essentially insulated, so as to exclude not only other undesirable girls but also boys, adults, teachers and researchers. Girls do not meet in large friendship groups and participate in a wide range of activities. Instead the most important aspects of the girls' lives are their best-friend relationship and their ability to attract and compete for boys (see McRobbie and Garber 1976).

Yet to explain girls' relative confinement to the private sphere of the home in terms of resistance is to overlook the much more obvious explanation that girls are conforming. If girls do not participate in boys' groups and their public activities and instead stay home listening to records with a close group of friends, this is not surely a form of resistance but, if anything, mere conformity to the expected feminine role which, by and large, is anticipated to centre on the home. Girls do of course go out and enter into social activities but, as we have seen, they do so on different terms from boys. For example, McRobbie argues that one reason the street remains taboo to women is made clear by the disparaging term 'street-walker'. The term 'street-walker' does not surely ban them from the street, but it does pronounce the terms on which they can be seen on the street, i.e., as girlfriend or slag. In other words, the girl's appearance on the street is always constrained by their subordination. The term slag is one of the ways through which this subordination is effected. This is why, rather than regarding girls' activities as a resistance, their participation in social life can be seen primarily as a product of gender subordination.

The researchers looked back at the 1950s and quoted Jules Henry who undertook a classic study of American teenage experience at that time. Henry found a similar tendency for girls to meet in small groups of friends:

As they grow towards adolescence, girls do not need groups, as a matter of fact for many of the things they do more than two is an obstacle. Boys flock, girls seldom get together in groups of four whereas for boys a group of four is almost useless. Boys are dependent on masculine solidarity within a relatively large group. In boys' groups the emphasis is on masculine unity; in girls' cliques the purpose is to shut out other girls (Henry 1963).

The representation of girls' friendships has not changed in many of the girls' weeklies. The messages and images of *Jackie*, analysed by Angela McRobbie (1991), depicted girls as never being able to trust another woman unless she is old and 'hideous', in which case she does not appear in these stories. Nor are friendships with boys depicted. The stories convey that it is impossible to talk to, or think about, a boy in terms other than those of romance. 'A favourite story in both picture-form and as a short story is the Platonic relationship which the girl enjoys. She likes him as a friend – but when she is made jealous by his showing an interest in another girl, she realizes that it is really love that she feels for him and their romance blossoms' (McRobbie 1991:101).

It was not until the women's movement of the late 1960s and early 1970s that solidarity among women was celebrated in the west, though in parts of the Third World it was far more prevalent. Amrit Wilson (1978) movingly describes the desperate isolation and loneliness experienced by Asian girls sent to Britain to be married. Those who came from joint families in India, Pakistan or Bangladesh to live alone with their husbands suffered most. She described the memories of Zubeida, a woman in her thirties who had come to England twelve years previously. What fun she had had with her friends!

On moonlight nights we women used to sit on the verandah and talk or sing and prepare and eat pan [betel leaf]. The busiest time of the year is the rice harvest, if the crop is good that is. There used to be a lot of work. I and other girls and women, we'd work the Dhenki, husking the rice or sometimes we'd go to the fields carrying tobacco and food for my brothers-in-law and cousins ... When I was a young girl I and my sisters, would get a boat and slip away, visiting friends from island to island. Of course the elders didn't like it. They thought we were tomboys but we loved it (Wilson 1978).

Johnson and Aries, who undertook one of the few extensive studies of adult female friendships in America, also stress the importance of talk:

The substance of women's friendships ... Close female friends converse more frequently than close male friends about personal and family problems, intimate relationships, doubts and fears, daily activities. Male friends, on the other hand, discuss sports more frequently than female friends. Adult women also report greater depth of discussion with their female friends about personal problems, family activities, and reminiscences about the past; men report greater depth in conversations with same-sex close friends about the topics of work and sports (Johnson and Aries 1983).

Deborah Lange (1988), who tape-recorded conversations between teenage girls, found that girls talk about relationships and boys talk about activities and plans. When girls and boys talk together she found they tend to take on male conversation styles and talk more or less the way boys talk.

Is Friendship the Same for Girls and Boys?

In popular culture girls' friendships are not supposed to last. It is usually assumed that friendships will be dropped when the girl gets a serious boyfriend, whereas boys are assumed to have friendships that last for life. Girls are more often integrated into the boyfriend's circle of friends, but it is unusual for boys to go out with the girl's friends, let alone become integrated into their network. Several questions spring to mind from this picture of female friendships: is it true that girls' friendships are invariably exclusive, or do girls have a broad range of friends, as boys do? What are the similarities between girls' and boys' friendships – indeed, do girls make friends with boys as well as girls? In what way does the structure of sexual relations affect relationships between girls and to what extent is competition for boys a crucial aspect of group life?

The first difference that struck me, in comparing the descriptions these girls gave of their friendships with McRobbie's and Henry's, is that although many girls had very intense friendships, they also participated in larger groups and knew a wide range of teenagers. As Lynn explains:

We know a lot of people who've got the same music
tastes, so if we go to a gig we meet people who we know
but not arranged to go with us. So we spend the evening
with them.

And Sasha:

You end up knowing a lot of people. Say you're in a
pub. Say you go round with a group and there's one of
the group that knows a lot of people and you get to
know them too. Then when you go out again you'll
know them too.

Or Alice comments:

Like, I've got friends at school but I've still got a lot
outside, so it really depends if I'm out with them or my
school friends. I'm glad I've got friends outside school,
'cos, like, spending days a week with the same people
gets really boring.

Some girls considered less intense and exclusive relationships were best. Becoming monopolized by an exclusive friendship was often mentioned as a problem to avoid. As Cheryl
explains:

I'm close to a lot of people now, not just with one person
in particular. I tried that out. I've had friends who you
like, see them every week or more often . . . But, like, in
the end you just . . . you just have to start lying and
pretend you're going to your dad's just to go and see
someone else just so as you can see your other friends.

It is the less intense and exclusive friendships that are most
appreciated, as Hannah confirms:

I can do what I like and she can do what she likes, and
we've got separate friends outside school and we've got
friends that mix with each other. So it's got big scope.
But also, she can ring me up and I can say, 'Oh, I'm
going out with so and so,' and she'll say, 'Oh, I'll see you
tomorrow then.' And there'll be no resentment. She
won't feel resentful or anything like that. That's what I
call a close friend. I can ring her up and talk when I'm
upset and she'll understand.

Claire mentions that one facet of closeness is being able to explain that you are doing something else or spend time with other friends and for this to be accepted.

The analysis of questionnaires gives support to the existence of networks of girls' friendships rather than to the exclusivity of their friendships. Where I asked girls to describe how many groups of friends they had, 67 per cent said they had two or more groups, and 33 per cent more than three. Most of these networks are quite large and most comprise three or more girls who all know each other and meet regularly. Other studies lend support to the important part peer groups play in girls' lives; even by the age of twelve or thirteen girls have groups of friends rather than one best friend. Other studies indicate that girls also participate in groups with boys and are an integral part of adolescent gangs, not just peripheral hangers on (see Wilson 1978, Smith 1978).

Nor do all girls prioritize boys, or could be said to be in competition for them. Some girls explicitly place friendship with other girls as more important than having a boyfriend. As Deirdre says:

> I think it's more important to have friends than, like, a boyfriend. I'd much prefer to have my friends, 'cos, I mean, I get on ever so well with them and we do a lot together, go and hear music, play music together and do all sorts of things.

Anne Campbell (1984), in her ethnographic study of girls' gangs in New York, found that by the 1970s the pattern of girls depending on male approval had changed, and that girls cared more about the opinions of their own sex. She suggests that this shift may be a result of a new interest in girls' behaviour in its own right, or it represents a real role change. In my research, some girls, as shown in the analysis of questionnaires, did not have boyfriends at all, and many had little contact with boys. The point I wish to make is that though some girls may compete for boys, this is by no means the main feature of their relationships. One reason why girls have been regarded as secretive and locked in exclusive groups is that researchers have encountered difficulties in interviewing girls. Some researchers were met with hostility when interviewing girls in a youth club where girls constantly made jokes among themselves. Rather than a result of the exclusivity of girl culture, it seems much more likely to be due to slight resentment towards researchers impinging on their leisure time. Or they may just have been having fun, 'taking the piss out of anyone they could find'. In my project girls were interviewed and group discussions took place during school time and provided a welcome diversion from classes. Under these conditions girls spoke freely and spontaneously about their lives. Girls' groups may be smaller and less fluid than boys' groups, but it is important to bear in mind that there is considerable variation and flux between and within girls' groups too.

If girls do have a wide range of friendships, is it true to say that their friendships are different in quality to boys', and is their participation in outside activities significantly curtailed? I shall first consider in what ways girls conceptualize their friendships and relationships with boys. Debbie, a black sixteen-year-old with two brothers, depicts the difference between girls' and boys' friendships in this way:

> The boys always try to act up to each other. They always seem to act tough. 'I'm more manly than you,' they say. Girls are much more sort of matey with their friends . . .

and the similarity:

> They both want to get their laughs and their kicks.

Having fun together is important, as Christine, a white, working-class girl from a single-parent family, describes:

> I think we found it giggly to go up to an old lady and say something to her and then run away. We went through a stage of knocking on people's doors and running away, that sort of silly game. I think it was 'cos we were bored. And all of us were making out we were getting on the bus or something and then make the bus

wait for us and then nobody got on ... You do it all the
time and you all know what is going to happen.

Amy describes fun in this way:

When you're having a joke, that is fun. Me and my
friends go out at the weekend. We just feel so sort of free
and without any compulsion to do anything, that you
could just be happy and be mad, just walk along the
street, happy and giggling and saying stupid jokes and
just laughing 'cos you're happy and it's just nice to be
free.

Apart from having fun, almost all the girls described their
close friendships as very intimate, where their innermost
thoughts could be aired:

I mean, you can talk to each other really well and when
you're upset they really are helpful. You come in the
morning and burst into tears and they just make you
laugh or they chat to you.

We never have real arguments. You sort of ring them up
and they're there and you can talk to them.

Your friends help you along. Like, I had trouble with
this boy, see, and, you know, something happened and
we started arguing and my friends helped me along in
proving him wrong. They always seem to give me the
right advice. I always take it and it always turns out
right.

These quotes illustrate the centrality of talk in girls' friendships. To speak about their experiences seems to be girls' main
means by which they handle the world. This is not to say that
girls just talk while boys act. But the overriding activity is
talking: what happened, who said what, who wore what, what
is going to happen.

Talk about boys [*laughter*], you do though, clothes,
records, where you're going – boys – what else do we
talk about? Girls we don't like – tarts.

Sexual reputation is a constant theme in girls' talk. Their
depiction of girls as slags or drags is just as intense as the boys'.

Girls describe talking as helping them 'sort out your mind', whereas when you are alone you get to feel 'desperate', 'depressed' and 'confused'. Talking to friends seems to be the main way that girls cope with the gossip and innuendo about their reputations and a way of defending themselves against unjustified insinuations. Seen in this context, no wonder the quality that is universally considered to be most important in friendship is trust and loyalty. Elizabeth describes a true friend as someone who will not repeat what is told in confidence:

> I probably trust her the most of anybody and she trusts me. I mean, of course people have told me things that they don't really want anyone else to know, and I've told someone else and everybody does that. But something that Jane tells me I couldn't tell anyone else. Something that I told her, I hope she couldn't tell anyone else.

She goes on to distinguish this from being close to someone, which does not necessarily involve trusting them:

> Like, Nicky and me are very close but I couldn't trust her at all. I don't think she could trust me either. We're basically not very alike. She doesn't really know how much something means to me when I tell her something, and, I mean, she's very bitchy behind my back.

Zoe has a similar concept of friendship:

> I think I just trust them in everything, the deepest secrets, every experience you've been through and it's just understanding both ways.
>
> If you tell on someone you'd probably be called a snide, you wouldn't have no friends left and they'll go round telling things about you that ain't true.
>
> Q *Called a what?*
> A snide. It means you tell someone something you're not supposed to tell, you promised not to.

Listening uncritically to your friend is a crucial aspect of the rapport. Many of the friendships the girls described had lasted almost all their lives – since they were two or three, or at least from primary school. This did not mean that everything could be shared, according to Tracy:

> There're always a few things which people keep com-
> pletely to themselves. But not much, 'cos I don't really
> have any problems which I can't tell anyone.

Other girls expected more than loyalty – sticking up for friends was important:

> To be on your side rather than someone else's – even if
> they don't agree. If you have an argument, your friend
> sticks up for you, even if she doesn't agree with your
> point, because she's your friend.

Maisie considered this extension of loyalty going too far:

> I think your mate should keep out of it if she disagrees.
> But if I really don't agree with one of my friends say, if I
> don't agree, I don't stick up for them.

Where to draw the line and risk a severe disagreement with a friend is a problem that fortunately does not arise very frequently, as friendship usually rests on a high level of consensus:

> Quite often if you're good friends there's a lot of things
> you agree on so it doesn't usually arise – a situation
> when you totally disagree with your friend.
>
> You can't argue with a friend.
>
> I mean, if you argue and they go off and they never
> speak to you again, they're not really a very good friend.

Being able to withstand a disagreement can be regarded as a facet of strong friendship.

Girls' friendships are characterized by loyalty and sticking up for your friends. The other side of the coin is bitching, which is constantly referred to as a female characteristic and as the source of aggravation often leading to fights among girls. Reading the girls' accounts, it is clear that girls fear that their friends may gossip. Girls are regarded as far more bitchy than boys, who are characterized as more straightforward and honest. This may be true but is likely to be a result of the

narrow tightrope a girl walks to maintain a reputation that
does not open her up to ridicule or ostracism. Bitching not only
refers to betraying confidences but typically involves calling
girls names and often casting doubts on their reputations.
Sexual abuse can be used in what is described as a joking way,
or more viciously:

> Friends are bitchy to each other in a joking way. We
> always keep calling each other names and we don't
> mean it.

So how can a girl tell whether or not to take the insult seriously?

> You can tell by their face, you can tell by the way they
> say it. 'Cos when we say it we sort of say something like
> 'You bitch' and start laughing, but then other girls just
> look at you or give you a dirty look, call you a name and
> walk off. They can't stand there and face you – they say
> it when they're walking past.

Bitchiness can also refer to friends talking about you behind
your back rather than to your face. Here bitchiness seems to
be a way of devaluing aspects of other girls that you wish to
signal as 'not you'. Sally describes this succinctly:

> Like, I am bitchy. I say, 'Oh, she's so fat.' You say it in
> front of friends, for instance, to see if they say, 'You can't
> talk, you're just as fat,' or to see if they agree with you.

A more vicious type of devaluing aspects of other girls is to
cast doubt on their sexual reputation, which is why much of
the bitching characterized by girls involved sexual abuse.
Jenny, for example, pinpoints what is meant by bitching in
this way:

> What people say when they bitch. They say they think
> some girl's a slag or something like that.

If rumours spread about you it can be unnerving, as Anna
comments:

> It undermines my own confidence to such an extent that
> I start feeling uncomfortable, then it bothers me. And if
> it isn't true, if it's false, it also annoys me. If no one has a

nice word to say about you, it's going to upset you. I
must say I get quite paranoid.

Judy had stopped going to discos because all the girls were
bitchy, shouted abuse at her and made her life a misery:

The main thing that comes to mind is 'Look at that
slag', or something like that ... I don't think most of
them know the meaning of the word really 'cos calling
someone a slag you've got to really have proof, haven't
you? I don't think it's very nice but it does upset you, it
starts me thinking that why are they saying it to me? I
don't go after boys all the time but I like to enjoy myself.

According to Denise, girls who want to have a boyfriend but
have difficulty attracting one are the most bitchy:

There's a group of girls who hang around together and
pretend they're not interested in boys but really are, like,
would really love a boyfriend but can't make the step.
They get a bit bitter and say, 'Look at that one, silly
slag.'

Bitching seems to be used as a way of putting other girls
down and differentiating the 'slags' from oneself – it is a way
of protecting one's own reputation. Other girls use the term
bitching to describe a betrayal of confidence, which is what
leads Cheryll to consider it unwise to share one's problems
with anyone:

You can't always trust friends ... Some of them talk
behind your back. You tell them something. That's why
you have to be careful who you hang around with, who
you speak to, 'cos even the slightest thing you tell them,
they can change what you've said and get you into a lot
of trouble. You might say something to them: 'Don't tell
anyone what I just told you.' The next moment the
whole school knows it.

There is an underlying contradiction here that friends are
defined as those you can trust, yet girls were also perturbed
that they could not always be trusted. This is not because
girls are any less reliable than boys but that they are in a

subordinate position vis-à-vis the boys who to some extent they are in competition for. The most risky confidences centre around sexual behaviour and feelings. One reason why so few girls talk even to their closest friends about sexual desire or actual sexual behaviour is through fear that their friends might betray them and gossip – spread the rumour that they are a slag. There is no parallel for boys to the risk of betrayal which can destroy a girl's whole social standing. Boys have less to betray in regard to other boys' confidences, as their reputations are not based primarily on their sexuality. They may agonize about whether their relationships are going well, but the social impact of their sexual behaviour is quite different. The slag categorization and constraints on a girl's sexuality act as a very effective way of restricting both the expression of a girl's sexuality and her freedom of action – her independence. The term poof or queer and milder terms such as wanker are used as slang but are not censures on the expression of sexuality in the way slag is.

Friendship among girls and boys is also significantly different in terms of the relation of friendship to the public or private sphere. Friendship for girls can lock girls more securely into the private sphere where emotions and personal life are the focus. Friendship for boys on the other hand is focused on the public sphere, where derogation and harassment of girls is a necessary tool for male superiority. Boys are more active together, and they dominate the public arena. Friendship groups, centred on the pub, nightclub, football game, cricket team or youth club are male dominated and girls can enter these arenas only on male terms. If boys have girlfriends, the girl tends to go round with him and is integrated into his friendships and even takes on his interests. A boy will be unlikely to tag along to any of the girls' activities or go out with a group of her friends. This boys' culture is a sexual culture, where sexual jokes and experiences are shared, songs sung and girls compared. For girls this sharing of experiences is only possible in the private sphere, or in the girls' lavatory.

Even the street is a male domain where a girl knows she can be attacked and is safer when in the company and protection of a man.

Getting a boyfriend often means integrating into his life. So inevitably girls very often drop their friends when they start to go out with a boy. There is an expectation that a girl will attach herself to his friends and his pursuits. Jeanette describes the process:

> Usually a girl will end up drinking in some pub that her bloke has always drunk in. Blokes – they'll always keep with their friends. That's one thing I've noticed. Blokes can go out and stay with friends whether they're going out with a girl or not, but if a girl's going out with a bloke, she drops her mates and then picks them back up when she stops going out with him.

Social life is now centred round boys and boys' activities – the pub is a male environment where girls may go with their boyfriend but do not feel confident to go on their own or even in a group of girls. This means that for boys their social life does not alter very much, whether they have a girlfriend or not – they are still welcome round the pub or can go on their own to a disco without the risk of being harassed or called a slag. There is a problem for a boy in becoming associated with girls' activities, as this could open him up to being categorized as feminine or a wimp.

Some girls describe their social life as restricted if they do not have a boyfriend, but certainly for working-class girls this is often connected with lack of money. Other girls have wide interests, and going out to pubs to hear bands and to discos is just as popular with girls as with boys. For example, Haylee says:

> Every weekend there are gigs. It's such a wicked atmosphere. It's terrific. Then there're parties at people's houses, or we go down the pub. At gigs you meet new people who've obviously got the same music tastes as you or they wouldn't be at the gig.

Other girls hesitate to go out on their own, and Greek and Asian girls are more restricted by their parents.

Some girls describe getting a boyfriend as important to overcome the hurdle of how to get back safely at night. As we shall see in Chapter 6, this underestimates the possibility of pressure and even encountering violence from boyfriends. It is often the boy who decides where to go, and when girls do go out they often go out with older boys. Even when they can afford it, girls are not always expected, nor sometimes allowed, to buy their round at the pub, indicating their subordinate status, and if challenged boys 'get the hump because they think it's degrading'. Buying a drink for a man puts a girl on more of an equal footing with him, which many men find hard to tolerate. This may be changing as girls, at least in some circles, may be more likely to be in work than young men. Some young women are developing strategies for resisting such pressures too. Haylee, a white, middle-class 'trendy', said:

> We go down the same pub most Fridays or Saturdays. The landlord's OK. We buy our rounds and then blokes buy us drinks.

Other girls described how they are ignored or expected to sit quietly while boys discuss how many girls they have made with their mates, often in the most explicit terms. This is how two girls described it:

> The boys you hang around with are mostly the same: like, they'll be talking about other girls all the time. They won't talk about what you've been doing, they just talk about what girls are bad and where they've been.
> Q *In front of you?*
> Yeah. Like, if you're sitting down and there's a whole crowd of boys talking about a girl, you'll be stuck there on your own and you say, 'I might as well go home.'
> They talk about some of our mates horribly, the ones they know, really good friends. They say they know for a fact that they are a slag because – say they're five of

them she's been passed around, then they'll talk about her. They say awful things anyway, whether it's true or not. Even when you're walking down the street they'll scream things at you.

Not all girls feel confident enough to challenge the boys' boasting, which is offensive to them. It humiliates them but they think it will cause trouble if they object. What is the boys' boasting about? The tendency of boys to boast in conversations with other boys was marked. Deborah Tannen (1992) in her analyses of men and women's conversations found that men frequently boast in public situations but women regard boasting as quite inappropriate. Boasting for men is about enhancing status, but for women it violates girls' egalitarian ethic, which emphasizes connection and similarity. Girls fear rejection if they appear too successful. 'Boys from the earliest age learn that they can get what they want – higher status – by displaying superiority. Girls learn that displaying superiority will not get them what they want – affiliation with their peers' (Tannen 1992:218).

Boys treat girls quite differently when they are with their pals, according to several girls:

They don't take any notice of you when they're with their mates. Or they take the mickey out of you.

A boy who would treat you quite reasonably or even be friendly with you when on his own, would treat you with disdain when with his friends, as Jenny describes:

We got a crowd round here near the flats. When they're with their mates . . . they're all hard and they call you all the names in the book. But when they're on their own they talk to you. They say, 'Hallo, Jenny, how are you getting on at school?' Or, 'I like your glasses.' But then when they're with their mates, it's 'All right goggles', and all the rest of it. That's what makes me sick. They're not like it when they're on their own. They only want to act big when they're with someone.

This behaviour, if shown by a girl, would of course be

described as 'being bitchy'. Since it is boys' behaviour, it does not get characterized in that way. No wonder many girls think pubs are one of the most boring places and prefer to be with their own friends.

The representation of female relationships is changing. One of the positive advances in women's fiction of the past decade, particularly black women's fiction, has been the placing of women centre stage and the positive depiction of female friend-ship. In *Sula*, for example, Toni Morrison (1974) portrays friendship between women as special and different, and argues that friendship had never before been depicted as the major focus of a novel. She portrays the love of Sula and Nel as far more valuable than Nel's love for her husband. It is not until too late, when Sula has died, lonely and rejected, that Nel understands the irrelevance of Sula's sexual 'infidelity' with Nel's husband and her own passion for Sula. More happily Alice Walker (1983), in *The Color Purple*, a bestseller and a Steven Spielberg film, depicts the possibilities of love between women, Celie and Shug, even when they are first presented as rivals for the same man's love. The depth and understanding between the two women is contrasted with the violence of many men's relationships with women. Again, as in *Sula*, the relationship between Celie, the oppressed wife, and Shug, her husband's lover, is far deeper and more meaningful than the relationship between men and women, which is depicted as violent and exploitative. Similarly Celie's protection of her sister Nettie, when she realizes that her stepfather who has sexually abused her throughout her childhood has similar designs on her, portrays women's ability to help others survive. These two books refute a common assumption that it is men that are all-important to women rather than the emotional ties between women. Finally, Audre Lorde's autobiographical account of her fight against cancer, *The Cancer Journal*, depicts friendship as a major focus of a woman's life (Lorde 1980). Publishing also now caters for teenage girls in providing them with a whole range of books where girl heroines are depicted as more independent and capable of friendship with both girls and boys (see for example Blume 1980).

Women's friendships are rarely represented on TV screens, and much of the programme content is saturated with sexist images of women. Standard humour is based on jokes directed at women. The 'mother-in-law' joke is a classic in the annals of (male) humour and 'the old cow reached heady levels of promulgation on worldwide TV in the 1960s and 1970s' (see Scutt 1990). Even feminist humour is often directed at women, women's bodies and women's bodily functions. Television is more often directed towards boys because they do not watch programmes planned for girls, while girls will watch programmes planned for boys (Carter 1991). In this way girls are inadvertently drawn into boys' activities. Soaps are an exception, and the popularity of *EastEnders*, *Neighbours* and *Brookside* may well be partly due to the positive representations of women and, in particular, female friendships. Detective serials such as *Cagney and Lacey* have also begun to show positive images of women colleagues. Mike Leigh's recent British film, *Life is Sweet*, is one of the first attempts to grapple with the reality of two sisters' lives and their resistance to marriage and conventional femininity, one through anorexia and the other through enrolling in a non-traditional apprenticeship course.

Girls from different ethnic groups form friendships and talk in similar terms about their experiences. Black girls I interviewed did not mention racist insults from other girls and boys occurring in school, but frequently referred to their experience of racist and sexist taunts outside the school. In school I did not find any expression of strong personal racism on the part of white girls towards black girls:

> The girls in school don't hang around in one group of coloureds, they sort of mix, they chip in. We've got one coloured girl and three white girls in my group and everyone gets on well together.

This is not however always so, and in one class the white girls in one friendship group, who were predominantly middle-class, tended to stick together. Some were aware that black girls were not in their friendship group. Tasha, a white girl, when filling in a questionnaire, answered the question 'In what way are you and your friends alike?' by writing, 'We are all white.'

Some of the white girls will challenge racism when they come across it in their friends, though, as in this example, to little avail:

> The other day it was a friend of ours got in an argument with a girl who had her cousin beaten up by coloured people and she said that she just couldn't stand coloured people and we said you should hate the people who did it but not just because of the colour of their skin or whatever. And she was really anti-coloured from then on.

Outside school some girls described antagonisms between groups of black and white girls. Jane, a white girl, is incensed about this:

> Some white girls called some black girls outside of school bad names – why they call them bad names I don't know. It's insane. Half of them don't even know what they're saying.

Paul, one of the white boys, described how black girls 'sent up' racist terms. Humour can be a way of subverting racism, of pouring scorn on such labels.

> A black girl might call another black girl a nigger, or she might call a white girl a honky, but it's light-hearted and done good-humouredly. They laugh about it.

I mentioned in Chapter 1 the awareness of dress differences as a key theme in the feelings of racial antagonism between black and white girls. Little is known about the importance of black style in creating identities among black girls. Almost all girls, both black and white, expressed strong interest in music, and most black girls preferred black music. In Ann Phoenix's (1992) recent work on race, class and gender in girls' friendships, fewer young white women than young white men shared the same music tastes with their black peers, which may be why young white women have fewer black friends than white boys.

There may also be another dimension to black and white girls' friendships. We have seen how the male world impinges on girls' friendships, which are often geared towards facilitating relationships with boys. The consequences of cross-race sexual relationships and their impact on friendship networks is in need of investigation.

Category Maintenance Work

Some girls do not only have different networks of girlfriends, but also know different sets of boyfriends. Jenny told me she finds it 'really hard to think of having a party, as so many people would come that it would be completely manic.' She is clearly anxious to keep her friends compartmentalized:

> I go swimming and I've known them since I was a baby and I grew up with them and they're just like my brothers. There are no girls there of my age ... Then there are my other friends, who might clash because of the lot at the swimming club. They're more pampered by their mums – like my mum calls the other lot ruffians – oh but they're not, they've just not been so pampered like the swimming club. They go swimming while the others would be in the pubs. I've got a mixture of friends. It's really hard if you're thinking of having a party and they might not get on.

Some girls describe friendship between girls and boys as no different from friendship within the same sex group. These girls thought it important to form a friendship with a boy before embarking on a sexual relationship. As Lucy explains:

> I think a boyfriend who isn't a friend isn't really worth having – it's best if you know them first, 'cos if you meet someone and it's, like, start going out with them straight-away, you don't really have time to develop a friendship. Whereas if you meet someone and you're just friends

with them before you start going out with them, then
there are things that you can talk about to a friend and
things which you talk about to a boyfriend, but when
these are combined, that's really best.

There is however a problem about forming non-sexual
friendships with boys. Bronwyn Davies in her study of
primary-school children makes two important points about
how gender differences are maintained in groups. Firstly, she
suggests that the dichotomy between male and female requires
collective activity to maintain it. This collective activity she
calls 'category maintenance work', which is primarily aimed
at maintaining the category as meaningful. Secondly, it is at
the boundaries of male and female behaviour that this category
maintenance work occurs. Girls and boys do not always behave
in sex-appropriate ways, nor do men and women. Often the
boundaries between male- and female-appropriate behaviour
are violated. This leads to a reaction to bring the deviant back
into line (Davies 1989:29).

Any deviant behaviour, therefore (for example a boy behaving like a girl), leads to other members of the group letting the
deviant know they have got it wrong. If a little boy bursts into
tears he is called a 'cry-baby'. If a little girl does the same she
is behaving just like a little girl should and she is comforted.
Teasing is often about bringing category deviants back into
line. Though individuals can deviate from the prescription of
masculinity and femininity, their deviance gives rise to category maintenance work, in order to maintain the category as
a meaningful one in the face of individual deviance which
threatens it. I came across many examples of this process.
Girls who behaved like tomboys and boys who did not boast
and liked to talk about relationships were teased and disap-
proved of by the more conforming group.

Jerry explains how some confusion could arise if you make
friends with girls:

Some of the time I like to hang around with girls more
than boys because they talk more sense about life and

everything. Lots of girls that I want to be friendly with take it the wrong way, and they think you want to go out with them, 'cos you're being friendly and having a laugh with them. They ask you out and you say, 'No, I don't want to go out with you. Sorry if I was leading you on. I just want to be friends.'

Antonio, an Italian boy, says:

I've got a lot of friends who are girls in school and a few where I live and I know a lot in Italy. They are different from the girls here because they socialize with boys more.

Hanging round with girls can give a boy a bad reputation, not for sexual prowess but for being gay. Witness the following discussion:

BOY 1 One boy in our school hangs around with almost all girls.

BOY 3 I think he's gay.

BOY 2 Does that mean I'm gay cause I hang around with girls?

Q *Why would somebody be gay if they hang around with girls?*

BOY 3 A lot of people say that.

BOY 2 That's just simple-minded people.

BOY 1 I don't like the idea of gay men, it makes me shiver.

BOY 3 With girls they don't mind gay men, but they hate lesbians.

BOY 2 I don't know any gay people personally and I don't think I'm as anti-gay as some people. The best explanation I've ever heard is that God made sex for two reasons, to reproduce and for pleasure, and if men only find pleasure with other men then let them do that.

Category maintenance work is more important for a boy than a girl as masculinity only reflects superiority if differentiated from femininity. It is an insult for a boy is to be called a 'woman'. I asked a group of working-class boys what calling a boy a 'woman' means.

MATTHEW It means a wimp. If you call someone a woman, he's a weed.

JOF Women are soft.

TOM He's weak. A weak person. You're a wimp if you can't stand up for yourself.

JOF If you let people boss you around.

MATTHEW Saying you're a poof is more insulting.

JOF I reckon Mike and Jim are –

TOM They'd say that was bad news.

MATTHEW No one likes to be called a queer.

JOF It's not natural.

We can see again how essential it is for boys to differentiate themselves from girls. To hang around with girls is to acknowledge their similarity. To be similar to girls is also to be associated with a lower status group, which means that it is far worse for a boy to show feminine qualities than for a girl to show masculine qualities. I remember the dilemma I was thrown into when my son, then aged five, insisted that he wanted to wear a dress to his rather straight-laced primary school. No such problem faces a little girl who wants to dress as a boy, but girls in some respects face a more contradictory situation. They are encouraged to behave in a feminine way, yet the attributes of femininity are generally considered inferior to masculine qualities. Parents and teachers are of course caught up with category maintenance work too, telling boys not to behave like sissys and girls not to be rough.

Yet the world is a contradictory place for boys as well as girls. Some boys, ironically, prefer talking to girls:

Some of the time I like to hang around with girls more than boys because they talk more sense about life and everything.

Jacky describes her relationship with her boyfriend in these terms:

We used to talk about everything really. Just everything you talk about to a mate you talk about to him. 'Cos I know him inside-out really. Every trick, like.

Other girls, however, have little or no contact with boys and few mentioned a boy by name when asked who they were friendly with.

Boys' Friendships

What emerges from boys' discussions is the way every topic is laced with masculine and feminine connotations, with either being 'hard' or 'soft'. Sport is hard, talk is soft. Girls said they were subjected to constant verbal sexual abuse – called slags, sluts, whores – while boys said it was sissy to talk to girls unless you are chatting them up. We have seen how boasting is a common characteristic of boys' interaction. Some boys found it sissy to talk about anything other than how to win and be on top. One boy found it difficult to describe anything he talked about with his friends other than football. To boast about how many girls you have made or to put someone down is 'macho' and 'tough'. Boys are pressured to act big in front of their friends. Their reputation is enhanced rather than damaged by sexual exploits, so the pressure is on them to 'mouth' – lie about how many sexual conquests they have made.

Some boys were different, talked about their feelings and were non-competitive and sensitive. But to avoid teasing and being accused of being 'wimps', they have to keep their heads down. Boys have to protect a 'masculine' façade of toughness, hardness and superiority. To call a boy a 'poof', a 'buttyman' (a term I had not previously come across, denoting homosexuality), is derogatory, but this term in denoting lack of guts suggests femininity – weakness, softness and inferiority. Boys are under pressure to disassociate themselves from anything female to 'prove' their masculinity. This often involves resorting to violence, as we shall see in Chapter 6 (Spender and Sarah 1980, Spender 1982).

Boys' attitude to fighting is a crucial facet of their friendships. Some boys keep out of fights if they can and work out which boys to avoid. Take Toby:

I could see how often people just started fights and then pulled knives out and I didn't want to get involved in that.

Q *What kind of boys don't you like?*

Maybe the kind of boy who is very babyish. And some of them get wound up too easily about things. One person is playing a game and he'll lose and then he'll sort of go mad and hit the table and whatever. He gets angry very easily.

In my interviews with boys, talk was given low priority by some boys but not by others. When I asked Danny, aged sixteen, what he talked about with his friends, he looked at me as though I was asking him a stupid question.

Talk, what do you mean?

When I pressed him about what boys talk about, he replied non-committally:

Dunno, football, I got a black belt. That sort of thing.

Q *What do you say if someone tells you they've got a black belt?*

I got a black belt too.

Other boys, like Jerry, an atypical sixteen-year-old, who wants to be a cartoonist and whose father is an actor, avoid fights and when Jerry was asked what he and his friends talked about answered:

Everything under the sun, famous people, sport, girls. What do you talk about? TV programmes, we compare families. Like if I know somebody's got a difficult family they talk about that all the time.

Abby, a friend of Jerry's, talked about trust being important too:

I'd tell Tony most things. I can trust him not to tell anyone.

Some of the girls think boys' friendships are very similar to girls', but that boys cannot admit to certain activities, such as talking. Typical of this attitude is Kay's view of talk as 'unmanly', something that girls do (girls' talk, gossip or chit-chat):

I think boys do talk as well. But they won't admit to talking the same as girls. I think boys aren't supposed to talk to each other, but they do. I mean, Kev has his mates round and may first talk and gossip the same as what girls do.

There is little doubt that on the whole boys' talk is different from girls' and much less focused on feelings and relationships. Though many of the boys I interviewed had been to primary school together, they often knew next to nothing about the home life of other boys in their class. Barriers appear to be particularly strong between the Bengali and white boys. There appears to be little room for negotiation or discussion when a dispute arises.

When I asked some Bengali boys what they do with their friends, they usually mentioned sport or other activities, going places and doing things. Rajam when asked what he likes to do at weekends replies:

Stay out as long as I want. Go do different things all the time. Go dancing. Go to parties. Go watch a video at your friend's house when their parents aren't there. When you've got a girlfriend you go out with her. When you ain't, you go out with your mates.

Mixing only with girls is however not an activity that Rajam relishes:

I once went to an old girlfriend of mine's party and it was just all her girlfriends. I was the only boy there. They were all just sitting around drinking lemonade and eating sandwiches. I don't like parties like that.

Q *What didn't you like about it?*

I knew them all from my old school but I just found it boring. It was more like a party you go to when you were seven and you're sitting round a table with paper hats on. Nah, not really. It's just that the light was on and their mum was bringing in trays of stuff and it was just like a girls' get-together. It was very exclusive.

Typically, boys found it difficult to talk about relationships with their friends; sport, activities and girls they fancy are the most typical topics of conversation. American football was called a 'sissy sport'. Boys have fun together, play sport, smoke dope. Boys seem to be posturing, vying for identities. Boys verbally play with labels denoting sexual or political identities – such as 'you're a commie [communist]', 'you're a sadist' – in a joking, teasing way, whereas girls' teasing is much more likely to be related to their sexual reputations or their romantic or sexual attachments.

In interviewing boys I did realize that I had underestimated the terms of abuse that boys throw at each other, but not their general association with femininity. To say 'Your mum is a slag' is considered very serious. It could break up a lifelong friendship. Jerry, who lives with his mother, a single parent, told me that his friendship with Alan had ended shortly after Alan's parents had split up. Alan had been a frequent visitor to his home, had often spent the night and they had been close friends. Their parents knew each other well. However Alan, upset that his parents were splitting up, for some unaccountable reason told Jerry that his mum was a slag, presumably because she was a single mother and had had a relationship outside marriage. Jerry had been so upset that he mentioned it to his mother, who had gone round to Alan's parents to have it out with them. It all ended badly and for the past year Alan and Jerry have not spoken. This incident shows how verbal sexual abuse can have material consequences, and be the source of breaking up relationships between adolescents as well as adults.

Several Bengali boys I interviewed vowed that if anyone cast aspersions on their mums' reputations, they would have no option but to fight. This is similar to South American and southern European cultures, where the worst insult is to say 'Go fuck your mother.' Such an insult is even worse than calling girlfriends slags. (A few years ago visiting a school I came across the insult 'Your father has AIDS', but this does not seem to be common any more.)

Boys are certainly under pressure to conform to what has been called 'hegemonic masculinity', that is, the dominant form of masculinity, even if this involves some degree of insecurity. Connell (1983:22) disagrees with this idea of masculinity as an impoverished character structure: 'It is richness, a plenitude. The trouble is that the specific richness of hegemonic masculinity is oppressive, being founded on, and enforcing, the subordination of women. Boys are well aware that they have many advantages.'

However, this type of hegemonic, macho masculinity contains within it a degree of violence that may be functional for capitalism but does not contain a 'richness', but an unfortunate connection with domination and militarism, as I shall show in the final chapter. It is also a significant aspect of the prevalence of violence between boys and between boys and their girlfriends.

How Different are Girls' Lives?

To depict girls spending most of their time at home, talking and listening to records, is incorrect. Girls do go out, though parents, realistically in view of the risks girls run of being molested, are more concerned about how girls are to get home and whom they are with. Girls frequently mention that their parents insist on their being home by a certain time. This does not, however, mean that girls do not go out. Many are out most nights, or at least most weekends – they visit pubs, gigs, discos, clubs and the cinema, and pursue a wide range of interests. Many play musical instruments (which incidentally makes one wonder why so few women play in orchestras and bands later on), go to football matches, go swimming, ice-skating, or hang around the flats, often in mixed groups of girls and boys.

Lesley Smith's 1978 study of a sample of delinquent girls who were active in such groups as Skinheads, Greasers and Hell's Angels indicates that some girls are also active in deviant subcultures. The girls she met participated in drugs, drink, sex, fighting and crime (see also Wilson 1978, Campbell 1984).

There can be little doubt about the seriousness of their group involvement, not only in social activity on the streets but in fighting, as shown in Cheryll's description of skinhead girls:

> You get them in a group and it's a power thing, they feel safe when they're in a group, and it's like the image of skinheads. I mean, I'm not saying that every single skinhead − of course not and probably most of them wouldn't demand your money or threaten you with knives − not if they were alone. But you get kind of pressganged into doing it when they're in a group.

Tracy describes how she 'bunked off' school with a group of boys and they'd break into cars and steal speakers and car radios or anything that was left in a car. This was 'good for a laff'. (She would only discuss this when the tape-recorder was turned off.)

Street fights are described by several girls. Some girls saw other girls as more of a threat than boys:

> I'm really scared of girls − walking down the road − girls will hit you where boys wouldn't. You know you can get away with a lot more with boys than you can with girls.

Some girls, like Sandra, describe quite violent incidents:

> I was walking home with Jenny, and these girls just started picking on us and everyone hit me and then they started hitting her. I went to help her and they started punching and mucking me about. It was out of order. I really hate that. They hurt me and cut me in the face. They booted me in the leg and Jenny was in tears. She had a mac on and a skirt. They ripped her mac and they gave her a bruise . . . There was no cause for it. We were only walking from school to the flats.
>
> Q *Why did they do it?*
>
> Just jealousy. I mean, she did look nice. If you had a

Burberry and it's expensive, ain't it? She had one of them on and 'cos they said to her, 'What do you think you're doing here?' She goes, 'We're walking through the flats.' And she didn't mean it but it sounded cocky, but she weren't. And they just went, 'You're not allowed to walk through these flats, this is our territory,' and things like that. They don't even live there but I do.

Frequently, how a girl is dressed and what her appearance conveys – her sexual attractiveness – seem to be grounds for a fight. How you look someone up and down can lead to trouble:

I had a fight with a girl. The way . . . she used to look at me as if I was real dirt. So I went mad one day and hit her. It gets me when they laugh at you. I think they've got a nerve. You go out and try and pay a lot of money for nice clothes and they go and sit there and take the mickey out of you. That gets me.

Another incident at a big conference on careers was described by several girls. Jane is fuming after it:

I can remember I had burns up my legs from having cigarette butts thrown at me and I walked out. I thought if I had a bomb I would happily drop it on them. I'm not prejudiced against anybody really, but that kind of thing I just hate. Fifteen- and sixteen-year-old girls who just don't know you and just make presumptions.

This is not to say that violence among girls is far less prevalent and far less a part of social relations than it is for boys. Only some girls participate in fighting, often the tomboys who are aping male behaviour. The antagonism between them is much more likely to be expressed verbally through 'bitching' than it is through physical fights. This will be explored more in the chapter on violence.

Conclusions

What generalizations can be made about girls' friendships? It is important to understand the mechanisms whereby relations between girls are dominated by gender, which governs the terms on which they enter into and participate in friendship groups. Female friendship can both protect and undermine girls in their social relationships. All girls stressed the importance of trust in their friendships. In a world in which a girl's reputation is constantly under threat both from girls and boys, trust is the most crucial attribute of friendship. A small group of close friends becomes essential in a world where other girls and boys will openly criticize you, talk behind your back, gossip about your every move and spread rumours. The primary demand in such a close group is trust and loyalty, but that trust is precarious. The gravest crime is to betray a confidence. The greatest risk is that confidence will be betrayed. Underlying this fear of breach of confidence is, I believe, the fear that your friend, with whom you shared your innermost feelings, may go off with your boyfriend. Nor is this fear a totally unrealistic one. This was the reason some girls maintained that other girls could not be trusted. The support of such a group is limited when girls are encouraged in all kinds of ways to prioritize relationships with boys.

Friendships among girls and boys have many similarities, but girls are still constrained by the lack of places for them to meet, the fear and reality of male violence and the constraints placed on them by parents. Though girls have a greater presence in the public world in pubs and other places of entertainment, they face the problem of how to get home unscathed. There are few places where girls can meet together without the danger of harassment. And girls are always subject to the fear of repercussions on their sexual reputation. Girls are not so much excluded from this world but enter it on different terms to boys.

The solution is to latch on to a boy and integrate with his network of friends. Boys sometimes obstruct girls' attempts to take part – attempts that often end up in girls blaming themselves for showing off or being pushy, behaviour that is related in some girls' eyes to acting like a slag. Conflict among girls, and bitching, are often less a matter of direct competition for the attention of boys than a defence of reputation, but at the same time reputation is defined in terms of behaviour conforming to the 'slag' label, a label that goes largely unquestioned but perpetuates the control of female behaviour by males.

These mechanisms surround the overriding predominance of sexual reputation as an ever-present force, censuring and constraining behaviour irrespective of the presence or absence of boys or whether the girls are in actual competition for particular boys. The language of sexual abuse censures girls even when boys are out of sight and out of mind. Such is the power of male dominance that its exercise is not dependent on the presence of the oppressor. In understanding the role this plays in determining the relationships between girls, I am reminded of the concept of power as 'self-carried' which has been elaborated by Foucault (1979), a power of male dominance which is not 'exercised' by boys over girls, but which girls carry with them and which enters into their lives and recreations. Boys are pressured to dissociate themselves from any activities or attitudes considered soft or female, as this would lead them to be associated with inferiority and weakness.

There comes a point at which the power of male dominance is felt to be directly exercised by boys and begins to break a girl's autonomy and her links with her own friends. This point is reached when a girl starts going out regularly with a boyfriend, where her own friendships give way to becoming integrated into the boyfriend's group, where she begins to be defined in terms of her relationship to him rather than to be her own person. In marriage it is she who will be expected to give second place to her interests and friends in favour of his networks and interests.

Anne Stafford (1991), who spent five months undertaking a study of teenage girls and boys, found a very similar picture. Solidarity among girls was strong and the girls created an autonomous culture to alleviate the boredom in the workshop. It was however a culture organized around boys, boyfriends, engagements and husbands. Their friendships, though close, were geared very much to finding a boyfriend, and it was understood that a relationship with a boyfriend would always take priority (Stafford 1991:107).

Even high-aspiring middle-class young women are not immune. A recent American study of predominantly white young women at university found that they responded to their shared vulnerability in the competition for boys, the 'sexual auction', not by teaming up to oppose it but rather by, at best, helping one another to fare as well as possible (Holland and Eisenhart 1990:108). The main problem was seen as finding a suitable man. The problem of finding Mr Right was accepted and women friends tended to be turned into a support group for finding him. Losing a woman friend to a man was not uncommon. A few girls were cynical about romance, but this was unusual.

For working-class young women, the possibility of maintaining friendships and interests is even more difficult. A recent study found that after cohabitation or marriage young women typically only spend time together talking on the telephone or on shopping trips, but have little opportunity to 'have fun' or go out. According to Pauline Naber's recent study of young women, they do not demand time for themselves and though they say they would love to go away on holiday together, rarely do so. Moreover, a great deal of the time they do spend together is spent sorting out their relationships with men rather than having a good time together. It can be argued that this is to avoid speaking directly to men about their dissatisfaction, which would cause too great an upheaval. Female friendship after marriage can therefore be seen to act as a way of consolidating unsatisfactory relationships with men (Naber 1992).

My own experience and the experience of many of the people I know confirms this. I have noticed that on the whole it is women who take on the man's interests on marriage. It is women's subordinate position in the marriage relationship that makes it difficult for them to maintain a life of their own and indeed many husbands oppose their attempts to do so. One problem is that there are few public places for women to meet that are not dominated by men. The public house, sports facilities, cafés, restaurants and youth clubs are all predominantly male domains. It takes a crisis like the miners' strike or a war to provide the opportunity for women to meet, and women have benefited greatly from these moments. During the miners' strike the ban on the movement of male trade unionists put women in a particularly powerful position. Films like *Thelma and Louise* have begun to depict women having fun together. Education is providing an opportunity for women to meet together and in my experience this often puts marriages under great stress. The husband of one of my students destroyed all her essays and another student told me how she had to read in secret; her husband threw out her books if he found her reading. There are outside pressures against women socializing together too. I remember when I went on a trip with two women up the motorway we were beset by men hooting and harassing us when driving. Women going out together are just not seen as respectable.

Adrienne Rich (1980), a renowned American poetess, was the mother of three sons who left her husband. She was one of the first to theorize about the importance of friendship. She argued that contrary to popular belief women's friendships with each other were often much closer than women's relationships with men, and rather than asking why women bond with other women, since their first love was their mother, we should rather be asking why it is that women prioritize relationships with men. In explaining this she argued that rather than such relationships just being natural, women are pressured into looking for fulfilment of their sexuality, emotional needs and economic support from men in marriage.

She argues that 'female friendship and comradeship have

been set apart from the erotic, thus limiting the erotic itself'. She puts forward the idea of a 'lesbian continuum' and argues that all women are by some definition lesbian, in so far as they have friendships with other women. There is a whole debate about what differentiates close relationships from erotic relationships. This idea of a 'lesbian continuum' has been criticized as 'expanding the category of the erotic to the point of eradicating the specificity of lesbian existence' (Modleski 1991:151). Lilian Faderman in *Surpassing the Love of Men* describes how in the last century it was quite acceptable for women to have intense relationships with other women; these would not be seen as unnatural or erotic. They were love relationships in every sense except perhaps the sexual (Faderman 1981:61). She suggests that today we are expected to deny such depth of feeling unless it is for a prospective or actual mate. This may be changing as more women leave unsatisfactory marriages. Two-thirds of divorces in Britain involve women petitioners. Liz Kelly (1988) describes how women who have experienced violence in their relationships with men often come to value their relationships with women. For some this represents a change in attitude, but for others it reflects valuing female relationships for the first time. Some women who live alone or with their children see their female friends as the most important adults in their lives.

While my research supports Rich's contention that women are pressured into relationships with men and their choice of friendships is heavily circumscribed, it indicates that some important changes are underway. Female friendship is gradually gaining recognition and some boys are valuing such feminine qualities as sensitivity and talk about human relationships. In the next chapter we will see how for most girls, at least initially, relationships with men replace their adolescent intimate relationships with other girls. They may have expected to be together for ever and ever, but these relationships give way to boyfriends, leading to cohabitation and eventually, when children are born, generally to marriage. There are strong ideological pressures on them to take this course. Some girls resist this pressure and do retain close friendships, but this is rare.

Bibliography

Beauvoir, S. de, 1952, *The Second Sex*, translated and edited H. M. Parshley, Penguin Books, 1972

Blume, J., 1980, *Are You There God; It's Me, Margaret*, Pan

Brittain, V., 1947, *Testament of Friendship: The Story of Winifred Holtby*, Macmillan

Campbell, A., 1984, *The Girls in the Gang*, Blackwell

Carter, B., 1991, 'Children's TV. Where Boys are King', *New York Times*, 1 May 1991, quoted in E. Runnels Ranck, 'The Meaning of Being a Girl', paper given at Alice in Wonderland Conference, Amsterdam, June 1992

Connell, R. W., 1983, *Which Way is Up? Essays on Class, Sex and Culture*, Allen and Unwin

Davies, B., 1989, *Frogs and Snails and Feminist Tales*, Allen and Unwin

Faderman, L., 1981, *Surpassing the Love of Men: Romantic Friendship and Love Between Women from the Renaissance to the Present*, Junction Books

Foucault, M., 1979, *The History of Sexuality*, Vol. 1, Allen Lane

Henry, J., 1963, *Culture Against Man*, Random House

Holland, D., and Eisenhart, M., 1990, *Educated in Romance: Women, Achievement, and College Culture*, University of Chicago Press

Johnson, F., and Aries, E., 'The Talk of Women Friends', *Women's Studies International Forum*, Vol. 6, No. 4, 1983

Kelly, L., 1988, *Surviving Sexual Violence*, Polity

Lange, D., 1988, 'Using Like to Introduce Constructed Dialogue: How Like Contributes to Discourse Coherence', Master's thesis, quoted in Tannen, D., *You Just Don't Understand*, p. 237

Lorde, A., 1980, *The Cancer Journals*, Argyle

McRobbie, A., 1991, *Feminism and Youth Culture: from 'Jackie' to 'Just Seventeen'*, Macmillan

McRobbie, A., and Garber, J., 1976, 'Girls and Subcultures: An Exploration', in Hall, S., and Jefferson, T. (eds.), *Resistance Through Ritual*, Hutchinson

Modleski, T., 1991, *Feminism Without Women*, Routledge and Kegan Paul

Morrison, T., 1974, *Sula*, Allen Lane

Naber, P., 1992, 'Youth Culture and Life World', paper given at Alice in Wonderland Conference, Amsterdam, June 1992

Phoenix, A., 1992, 'Race, Social Class and Gender in Girls' Friendships', paper given at Alice in Wonderland Conference, Amsterdam, June 1992

Rich, A., 1980, 'Compulsory Heterosexuality and Lesbian Existence', *Signs* 5(4), pp. 641–60

Scutt, J., 1990, *Even in the Best of Homes*, McCulloch, North Carlton Victoria

Smith, L. S., 1978, 'Sexist Assumptions and Female Delinquency: An Empirical Investigation', in Smart, C., and Smart, B. (eds.), *Women, Sexuality and Social Control*, Routledge and Kegan Paul

Spender, D., 1982, *Invisible Women*, Writers and Readers Press

Spender, D., and Sarah, E. (eds.), 1980, *Learning to Lose*, Women's Press

Stafford, A., 1991, *Trying Work*, Edinburgh University Press

Tannen, D., 1992, *You Just Don't Understand: Women and Men in Conversation*, Virago

Tiger, L., 1969, *Men in Groups*, Thomas Nelson and Sons

Walker, A., 1983, *The Color Purple*, Women's Press

Wilson, A., 1978, *Finding a Voice*, Virago

Woolf, V., 1929, *A Room of One's Own*, Harcourt

Chapter 3
Love and Marriage

I want to get married to make kids legitimate. But in a way you don't
want to get married because marriage has gone out. You might as
well suit yourself (Tania, aged sixteen)

If you don't want to get married and want to live a free life . . .
everyone will call you a tart, like you've got to go out with a bloke for
a really long time and then marry him (Leah, aged sixteen)

Within popular culture love and marriage are assumed to
provide us with the most fulfilling experiences of our lives.
With religion in decline, families breaking up and people
leading more isolated, fragmented lives, the ideology of love
and marriage is still alive and well. In popular discourse, in
song, in the arts, love is conceptualized as overpowering. You
can be 'swept off your feet' and fall in love 'at first sight'. It
can happen like 'a bolt from the blue'. And it lasts for ever
and ever and embraces mind, body and soul. It is an illusion,
but this does not dissolve the myth. The whole idea of romantic
love expresses a yearning for meaningfulness, a yearning for
stability, for a world in which women and men understand
each other and love each other. The assumption that love is
'natural' and 'just happens' also makes the romantic myth
very difficult to contest. It is at some level pleasurable.

The nuclear family for all its strengths embodies a fundamental weakness. It is based on inequality, organized around the
unpaid and often unacknowledged labour of women within
the context of a male-dominated society. The woman gives up
her name, her previous identity, and as we have seen is
expected to be integrated into her husband's interests and
networks. In this chapter I investigate how girls and boys view
marriage and illustrate how the way masculinity and femininity

were traditionally constituted is no longer functional to the economy, and how new forms of femininity and masculinity are developing, in the latter case with dire effects. Behind the myth is a different reality. For men, at the extreme, it legitimizes so-called 'crimes of passion'. A hundred women in Britain and a thousand in the USA (Jones 1991) are killed per year by their spouses or boyfriends, often after years of beatings.

Girls on the whole do not subscribe to the illusion of living 'happily ever after', and are increasingly aware of the inequality that lies behind the romantic myth. They express a contradiction in their views of marriage which at first I found difficult to understand. On the one hand they reject a romantic view of marriage and see marriage realistically as rendering them unequal and subordinate. On the other hand they do not see any alternative. As Mandy says, 'The girls who didn't want to get married are lezzies and the boys who didn't are queer.' In this chapter I explore what girls mean by love. Love legitimates sexual expression and steers female sexuality into the only safe place for its expression, in cohabitation and marriage. The romantic view of married life is waning, as can be seen in girls' magazines, recent fiction and the girls' own experience. Divorce in Britain has increased fivefold since the 1960s, a higher increase than in any other European country; currently one in three marriages will break down. Half of the girls in my research were no longer living in intact families.[1]

Drawing on my interviews I show how girls adopt four strategies to deal with the contradiction between the realistic and the romantic view of marriage. Some girls deny there is any alternative; some postpone it for as long as possible; others delude themselves that finding the 'right man', the Prince Charming of their dreams, will save them from their mothers' fate. Lastly, some girls avoid marriage by cohabiting and see marriage as necessary only 'for the sake of the children'. In contrast to the grim picture of marriage, the years before marriage are envisaged as providing an opportunity to have fun, to travel and to have a career rather than merely a job. Increased choice to have sex outside marriage, to pursue a career, to have children outside marriage may not, without changes in the wider social structure, make life easier for girls.

For boys marriage is far less contradictory. Most boys see marriage, if they think about it at all, as providing them with someone to look after them, who will be faithful and gentle (i.e. obedient). A few boys are in favour of equality and sharing childcare, but overall boys' ideas about girls are traditional and reactionary and have not kept up with the changing climate.

The Function of Love

As we saw in Chapter 1, the construction of sexuality involves the construction of differences between slags and drags: a certain kind of sexuality − essentially promiscuous/dirty in nature − is not 'natural' for all girls/women, but only resides in the slag. Yet non-slags are always viewed as possibly available, potential slags, until tried and found to be drags or possible wives. In other words, there is always a blurring of the two categories. It is not easy to make the distinction, despite the apparent essential differences, since the status is always disputable, the gossip always unreliable, the criteria always obscure. So what marks the difference? The presence of love. Deirdre Wilson, in her study of delinquent girls carried out in the late 1970s, also found that love is crucial to rendering sex a legitimate activity: 'The fundamental rule governing sexual behaviour was the existence of affection in the form of romantic love before any sexual commitment. For most of the girls, love existed before sex and it was never a consequence of sexual involvement' (Wilson 1978:70–71).

She goes on to note, however, that 'Given the threat of rejection [for sex without love] it was difficult to discover just how many girls actually believed in the primacy of love, and how many simply paid lip-service to the ideal. Nevertheless, the fact that the girls found it necessary to support this convention, whether they believed it or not, was an important fact in itself' (Wilson 1978).

Nice girls cannot have sexual desire outside love. For them sexuality is something that just happens if you are in love, or, if you are unlucky, when you are drunk. Girls must be on their guard against being taken advantage of. If this happens the general consensus of opinion is that it is the girl's fault:

> It happens a lot. But then it's the girl's fault for getting silly drunk in the first place that she can't, she doesn't know what's going on or anything.

Love or 'falling in love' is therefore both a denial and an expression of sexuality:

> I used to fall in love with pop stars, now I fall in love with people. When you're in love you ain't got no problems.

The upsurge of excitement at the sight of the object of love/ desire is surely sexual but, significantly, it is not recognized as such by the girls: 'Within these groups of girls, expressions of sexuality could only receive support or be condoned when they maintained the triangular relationship of love, sexuality and marriage' (Wilson 1978:71).

Everyone talks about love and young girls are expected to fall in love but it is unclear exactly what love is. Julia Kristeva, a French analyst, expresses the ambiguity: 'We were trying to decide if, when speaking of love, we spoke of the same thing and of what thing? When we said we were in love, did we reveal to our lovers the true purport of our passions? We weren't sure, for when they in turn declared themselves in love with us, we were never sure what that meant exactly, to them' (Kristeva 1989:2).

We usually assume we know what we mean when speaking of love. Since the girls I interviewed spoke of love, I tried to discover what exactly they were referring to, and to what extent these meanings were shared. Few girls were clear about what being in love entailed, although invariably love was given as the only legitimate reason for sex. Girls often changed their minds about whom they loved when sexual desire appeared to be what was really being alluded to:

> You think you're in love and then when it finishes you find someone else who you like more and then you think the last time it couldn't have been love so it must be this time. But you're never sure, are you, 'cos each time it either gets better or it gets worse so you never know.

> You think you're in love loads of times and you go through life thinking, 'God, I'm in love,' and you don't do anything. You want to be with this person all the time. Then you realize you weren't in love, you just thought you were . . . I thought I was in love and then I went away and when I came back I realized I wasn't. It wasn't love at all. So I finished it and I was much happier.

This could be interpreted as the expression of sexual attraction rather than anything more complicated. Some girls said they had 'been in love loads of times', whereas others said they 'had never really experienced it'. There was a good deal of discussion about how long it took to fall in love. Some girls talked about 'love at first sight', others thought it only happened gradually:

> It takes a while to happen. I mean, it sort of dawns on you that you finally love this person. Don't think it happens straightaway. I mean you might say, 'Oh, look at him, I love him, I think he's really nice,' but you can't really say that until you know him really well.

Given this ambiguity about what love involves, it could well be that love is used as a rationalization after the event for sleeping with someone, rather than, as Wilson suggests, as always existing before sex could occur. The confusion that girls experience over whether or not they are in love arises surely from sexual desire. Love is supposed to last for ever or at least for a long time, and is the main reason that girls give for getting married. The distortion of what is really sexual desire into 'love' means girls must find it difficult to separate their sexual feelings from decisions about marriage and long-term commitment. As Eileen said,

> Girls have got to keep quiet about sex and think it's something to be ashamed of.

However it is quite legitimate to talk of love.

It is also legitimate to express desire for pop stars. Pop stars infiltrated girls' magazines in the 1980s to such an extent that according to McRobbie (1991), 'It is pop rather than romance which now operates as a kind of conceptual umbrella giving a sense of identity to these publications.'

She attributes the decline of *Jackie* magazine and the rise of *Just Seventeen* and *Smash Hits* to a rejection of romance as a cultural phenomenon and its replacement by far more overtly sexual fantasies of real-life pop stars. Instead of romantic stories where women are often depicted in a passive, subordinate way, these romantic narratives are being replaced by excessive interest in pop stars and celebrities who increasingly provide the fantasy material. The emphasis in these new magazines is on boy stars who have replaced the fictional boys found in magazine stories. *Jackie* was not able to plug into the celebrity network and lost its sales to *Just Seventeen*. McRobbie argues that this signposts 'the end of romance'. Romance, according to *Jackie*, was one of the hallmarks of femininity. But femininity is changing. Now a more dynamic image of femininity is being presented, mocking and slightly ironic, implying a degree of distance rather than slavish subordination.

Pop-star images give girls the opportunity to explore sexual feelings from a safe distance. Infatuation with a pop star is a way of directing sexual feelings which are unacceptable if expressed directly. Cora, a white sixteen-year-old girl, explains:

> There're always sort of film stars or people on TV or pop singers that girls get infatuated with. You can accept more that it's never going to happen, that it's just nice.

> Nice to be able to look at somebody and think how
> wonderful they are. Otherwise it's not a very cheering
> world. It makes my world go round.

These magazines give girls an opportunity to look at pin-
ups of boys and reflect on what boys' bodies are like without
being confronted with thinking about sexual involvement.
There are also degrees of sexual pleasure in viewing such
representations. The images are often full length and emphasize the male body as sexual as well as having 'dreamy' good
looks (see McRobbie 1991:171). This is a marked shift from
the 'romantic' stories which were typical of girls' magazines
such as *Jackie* in the 1960s, where female passivity and traditional sex-role stereotyping were emphasized. A strong image
of femininity can be seen on TV soaps such as *Grange Hill*,
Neighbours, *EastEnders* and *Brookside*, which present women as
less romantic and as strong if not stronger and more independent than the men.

Heightened sexual interest and falling in love appear to be
interchangeable, as Eileen suggests:

> I mean, one minute you think he's nice and then the
> next minute you'll think he's really wonderful and want
> to be with him all the time – you begin to see him in a
> different light.

Some girls see 'falling in love' as transitory:

> I've got a couple of friends who are fifteen, and they say
> they're in love but I don't know if I'll ever be in love. I've
> had boyfriends and I don't think I've actually . . . I mean,
> the whole sort of having to live with him every day of my life
> would drive me mad. I think love's, like, a bit of a
> complicated thing. I think there's lots of kinds. There is love
> that is more infatuation, where it's completely give every-
> thing. Just sort of wide-eyed. Then there is love when you
> are able to trust someone. You'll both be on equal terms . . .
> But to live with some . . . I mean, if I go and stay with
> friends for, say, three days, by the end I've had enough.

Yet still the only really safe place for the expression of

female sexuality is in a long-term relationship, usually leading to marriage. The 'legitimacy' of love is precisely its role in steering female sexuality into the only 'safe' place for its expression. The result is that a girl either suppresses her sexual desire or channels it into a steady relationship. The extent to which young heterosexual women define sex in terms of love, romance and relationships with men leads to a widespread acceptance of defining sexual practices in terms of men's needs, to the neglect of women's.

McRobbie (1978, 1981) originally argued that girls elaborate romance as resistance to the harsher social realities of school and work. Yet she did not locate this romance within a male-dominated culture and peer group. My analysis suggests that romance is part of the oppressive sex gender system, not some celebratory culture of resistance developed in response to an oppressive culture. As Germaine Greer so aptly put it in *The Female Eunuch*, 'The first kiss ideally signals rapture, exchange of hearts, and imminent marriage. Otherwise it is a kiss that lies. All very crude and nonsensical, and yet it is the staple myth of hundreds of comics called *Sweethearts, Romantic Secrets* and so forth' (Greer 1971:172).

Contrary to the popular myth, romance is not unrequited love as in the medieval ballads, but the narrow route to marriage. Nancy Chodorow, referring to clinical and sociological evidence, concludes, 'Most of these studies argue . . . that women's apparent romanticism is an emotional and ideological response to their very real economic dependence' (Chodorow 1978:197). She suggests that women are less romantic and have acquired a real capacity for rationality and distance in heterosexual relationships.

Recent research on women students attending American universities corroborates the view that romance is not so much resistance as conformity. Holland and Eisenhart (1990) summarize their findings regarding the privileged position of men and boys in peer groups which they argue was constructed from the long-standing tradition of romantic love:

The face of patriarchy most directly confronted the women in the world of romance and attractiveness. School and college peer cultures insist that a woman's social worth, her social prestige, is mostly a function of her sexual attractiveness. Hence gender relations are serious business for a woman, not only because of the ultimate economic and social importance of marriage, but also because her sexual attractiveness is so immediately emphasized in the peer culture she participates in during her school career (p. 218).

They concluded that though romance as opposition does occur at times, it is likely that it usually co-exists with a peer-run system of male privileged gender relations that draws on the same tradition. Both in my research and the American study, decreasing involvement in schoolwork coincided with increasing investment in romantic relationships. It seems that oppositional youth groups are more likely to develop in response to class, race and age hierarchies than in response to gender hierarchies.

Tania Modleski (1991) makes a similar point when she suggests that the popularity of romances is a cross-cultural phenomenon, and romances provide a common fantasy structure to ensure women's continued psychic investment in their oppression. The promise of heterosexual love ensures the impossibility of women ever getting together to form a subculture and hence develop a system of values that will effectively challenge and undermine a hegemonic patriarchal ideology. Perhaps Margaret realizes the illusion of love when she says:

> You think you are in love with a person but sometimes you're just in love with the idea of being in love . . . Sometimes when you fall in love . . . You don't see the point of it any more, you don't get anywhere . . . and you forget about the one you're supposed to be in love with.

Views of Marriage

I don't want to get married until I've had my life (Marianne).

This comment by Marianne is typical of the unromantic realism about marriage expressed by many of the sixteen-year-olds in this study. At sixteen Marianne is a very lively girl, out most nights, and brimming with plans for the future. She wants to be an actress and go round the world. A year later she is an assistant at Woolworth's, hardly ever goes out and is saving to get married. All her ambitions for her future have dissolved and she has given up any ideas of a career. In a year or two she will be married, with two children and a future of part-time low-paid work ahead of her, locked in a subordinate position in the family.

Terry Jordan interviewed seven women who were brought up in the 1950s and poignantly describes how girls at sixteen were only concerned with marriage:

When I was in my last year at school, I think – and this is speaking from the point of view of most of the girls in my class to hear us talk – we wanted to get married. That was the be-all and end-all. Most of it, I realize now, was that we wanted to experience sex; we really were curious about it. We also wanted to get shot of those tyrannical parents of ours . . . As far as sex went, I was simply told never to do it! . . . It was easy to say 'No' in those days because it was expected you would, that was the beauty of it (Jordan 1990:4).

Similarly, Pearl Jephcott (1942), who carried out a pioneering investigation into the lives of girls aged seventeen to twenty-one in the 1940s when no equivalent work existed, found that two things dominated their lives: first, their homes, and second, the extent to which future marriage appeared to occupy their thoughts throughout adolescence. Practically every girl said she wanted to give up her job when she got married. None thought her job was more important. Many of the girls I interviewed in the 1980s, on the other hand, talked in terms of careers as a way of delaying the inevitability of marriage and in terms of working after marriage, combining careers with marriage.

Not that marriage is not still at the back of their minds. When Diana Leonard in her research in Swansea in the early 1970s asked girls when they had decided to get married, they said they could not remember a time when it had not been a consideration. Any relationship without marriage in mind was unimaginable. Rather than choosing not to get married, girls fail to get married (Leonard 1980). Sue Sharpe (1976) in her study of over 200 girls from the fourth forms of four schools in Ealing in the 1970s found too that 82 per cent of them wanted to marry – a third of them hoped to get married by the time they were twenty and three-quarters by the age of twenty-five. They accepted that a husband and family were the most satisfying things in a woman's life.

The girls I interviewed in the mid 1980s were either unaware or embarrassed to talk about sex openly. They still saw marriage as eventually inevitable, though cohabitation before marriage was preferred by a number of girls. In 1979–81, over a fifth of women marrying had cohabited with their husband beforehand. In the last decade cohabitation before marriage has almost become the norm. In 1987 nearly half of all women who married had lived with their future husband before marriage.

This study was carried out in an inner-city area in London where the rate of family breakdown is rather higher than the national average. Fifty-two of the sample filled in a questionnaire about their family circumstances. Over half of these, thirty-two, were still living with both parents. Of the remainder, fourteen were living alone with their mothers (one of these was a widow), three lived with father and stepmother. The prevalence of marriage and the tendency of divorced couples to remarry is usually interpreted as lending support to its success in providing couples with a secure and romantic future – the 'they lived happily ever after' of fairy-tales. What is left out of this picture is that for young people there is little alternative to marriage even if preceded by cohabitation.

Active sexuality is only rendered safe when confined to marriage and wrapped in the aura of love. This is one reason why feminist critiques of marriage and the family have not met with popularity from most women who see feminism as threatening their commitment to husbands and children. Marriage is seen as essential for economic reasons. For young women, marriage represents economic and cultural security as much as if not more than wages.

Realism about Marriage

Divorce, in view of its high rate, was sometimes put forward as a reason for avoiding marriage, though it rarely led girls to discard the whole idea:

> If you look at our homes, it's not such a good idea – there's so many people's parents who are divorced. It's about 50 per cent of marriages fall apart.

Girls whose parents had separated often expressed distress:

> It happened to me not last November but the one before. I live with my dad now. They just decided to separate and we worked it out. But for about a month I walked around crying, even in lessons.

> You feel really unwanted. You feel like, 'Oh they don't care about you. They just care about what they feel themselves.' I felt so depressed because, I dunno, it's the sense of failure.

Feeling uncared for is a constant theme:

> My parents got divorced when I was about two and I've always felt they don't care about me. They just care about themselves. I always think people are against me. It's horrible.

Others accept divorce with greater equanimity: Deborah puts her mother's failure at marriage down to her lack of interest in housework:

> My mum's been married twice, once my first dad left

when I was about three, but that wasn't – I mean, none of the marriages have been bad, sort of 'taking to court' sort of relationships. You have to go to court but they've always been decisions made together. It's just that my mum, my mum is so untogether about housework, she really wasn't made to be married. She's much better off by herself. I'm more sort of together about housework and money and things. She's terrible with money and it's caused problems with my second dad because he was quite the opposite and it caused a clash. I still go to my second dad every two or three weeks and we get on fine. I'm going on holiday with my first dad and his wife and my friend Jo. We get on all right too . . .

Overall the girls' view of marriage is not romantic but seems to be realistically based on their observations of the marriages of their own parents, relatives and acquaintances. Yet their views are contradictory. Girls rarely speak romantically about marriage, but often describe it as bringing subordination and loneliness. Despite this, most of them see themselves eventually getting married. Girls are well aware of the falseness of the romantic image but still hanker after meeting Prince Charming and living happily ever after. According to Jessie Barnard (1973), it is the discrepancy between the ideal of marriage as fulfilment and the grim reality that women encounter that emerges as depression and despair later on. She argues that married women have higher rates of depression, mental breakdown and drug dependency than any other section of the community. Other studies have painted a similar picture. In their study of women with young children living in the borough of Camberwell in London, Brown and Harris (1978) found that two-thirds of married women with a child at home suffered from clinical depression or were borderline cases, compared with 17 per cent of a cross-sample of all women in the study. Married working-class women had a higher risk of depression when they had young children at home. Husbands are not likely to recognize the difficulties of childcare, which they see as a cushy job. This trivializes the women's work and lowers their self-esteem.

There is evidence that men benefit much more from marriages than women. Single males are four times as likely to be in mental hospitals than are married males of the same age. Married men are also healthier than married women and single men. For men, marriage offers material advantages which the boys recognize. As Spike in Paul Willis's study says:

I've got a right bird. I've been going with her for eighteen months now. Her's as good as gold. She's fucking done well, she's clean. She loves doing fucking housework. Trousers I brought yesterday. I took 'em up last night, and she turned them up for me. She's as good as gold and I wanna get married as soon as I can (Willis 1977).

In contrast, girls describe marriage as offering no such material advantages, but rather a greater burden of domestic labour. The modern view of marriage encompasses ideals of equality and sharing, but there is little evidence that these have led to a greater division of housework and childcare among married couples. Even among middle-class couples, where greater equality could have been expected, the evidence suggests that men have changed very little.

Girls are realistic about the constrictions of marriage. Marianne's view that she would get married 'when I have had my life' is shared by others. Frequently girls refer to 'having fun', 'travelling the world' and 'doing what I want' before settling down. 'Having one's life' seemed to refer to being able to decide what you want to do without consulting others. Girls see children as a heavy responsibility. Marriage they describe as a domestic burden that carries little in the way of reward, accompanied by a financial dependency that can be both a constriction on the mother and a bone of contention between husband and wife:

My dad won't give in, like. My mum, she sort of goes short now and again and she asks him for extra money, and he just won't give it to her. I think other families are like that. If you don't have to rely on a man, they don't feel so tight with their money.

Above all else the girls recognize the isolation of being at home:

> My mum hates being at home, you know, but she had to stop working because she's going into hospital and she's going to hate that – she is going to be so bored.
>
> Q *Is that why she works?*
>
> Yes, she just don't like being at home.

Girls do not accept that domestic work is woman's role and a number of girls express strong disapproval of the way their mothers are treated. Girls are aware that their mothers often suffer treatment from their husbands that no employer would get away with.

> My dad thinks she should be a total wife/mother image, be there, ready and waiting. The meal should be ready and if he clicks his fingers, she should go running.

Girls are aware of the power relations in marriage and a number were adamant that they would not put up with being bossed about:

> I don't want to have people bossing me about, telling me what to do. And that's partly why I don't want to get married, 'cos I think that it's a sort of tie to you, to get married. From the experience of my mum and dad getting married I just don't think it's a very good thing.

Beatings and cruelty are also referred to and several girls describe the boy they would marry as one who 'does not beat [them] up'. Sandra thinks beatings are usually associated with drinking:

> Q *Is it common for men to come home drunk?*
>
> Yes, it's like this lady round our flats, she gets beaten every night because her husband goes drinking, comes home about twelve, starts beating her, you know, for nothing, saying she's been out with this man, she's done this and done that, he just makes it up, any lies and starts trouble.

Or as Mandy says:

> The one thing I don't like men doing to their wives is
> beat them up. At least that's what it's like with the next-
> door neighbour. She's married and they're her children
> and her husband when he comes home at night, he beats
> her just for the fun of it and then he wants to go to
> bed with her afterwards ... I don't want that if I get
> married.

Some families face other severe problems – Barbara describes
how her father, who was at one time a psychologist, had
frequent nervous breakdowns which meant her mother not
only had to work full-time but also had to look after him
through his breakdowns:

> It must be awful to think that you've wasted your life
> getting married to somebody like that. She's just stuck
> with him now and forever unless he gets better or gets a
> great deal worse and has to be taken into hospital.

Girls are remarkably clear about the grimmer aspects of
woman's lot in marriage. As Sandra puts it:

> The wife has to stay at home and do the shopping and
> things. She has got more responsibility in life and they
> haven't got much to look forward to ... We've got to
> work at home and look after the children till they grow
> up, you've got to go out shopping, do the housework and
> try to have a career. The man comes in and says 'Where's
> my dinner?' when we've been to work. They say, 'You
> don't work.' It's because boys are brought up expecting
> us girls to do all the work. They expect their mums to do
> it and when they get married they expect their wives to
> do it. They're just lazy.

Their views on marriage were based on observation of their
parents and the unfair division of work between husband and
wife:

> My dad won't do anything, he won't make a cup of tea,
> he says he does the work for the money and the rest is up
> to my mum – she does part-time work.

Some girls are critical of their mothers for not resisting more. Belinda's parents had separated some years before:

> I think my mum was a bit of a mug. She let my dad do nothing and then when he realized that she wasn't there to do everything and she asked him to do things he got obstreperous and they split up. He thought men are there to sit and enjoy themselves and women are there to work. It was impossible to change him. By then it was too late.

The growing number of women in the labour force has had little effect on increasing the involvement of men in housework, and girls are very aware of this. Sylvia is critical of how hard her mother works:

> She works too hard. She gets up at half-six in the morning and works till eight, and then goes to work at nine to seven at night. I just wouldn't be able to do that. Then she works all weekend . . . She's quite successful in what she does. But she does so much work, I probably won't be able to do that.

Girls' expectations of boyfriends and marriage are often not very high and are as much about avoiding an inappropriate boyfriend as finding a suitable one. So Maggie says:

> I don't expect very much, because most of them [boys] aren't very bright and some of them are on the dole. I just don't want anyone who hasn't got a job and who just thinks about going to bed with you and leaving you.

When asked what kind of a husband she would like, Maggie said:

> Not a sexist. Some men seem to define different jobs like, these are for men, these are for women. Women have to stay home and go out to work and do all the jobs in the home and they [men] come home and say, 'The wife doesn't do anything.'

Jane wants

> Someone who's lovely and not sort of sexist.

Mothers warn their daughters about boys in no uncertain terms. Roxana, an Indian girl, explains her mother's view:

> She would tell me off 'cos she don't trust boys. It's not that she don't trust me, she don't trust boys. She knows what they're like, as she has been through all that, she goes, 'It's not worth trusting them.'

Or as Haylee puts it:

> My mum told me never to go with boys because they're bad and they damage your health. She says they ruin your life if you get pregnant. She says it's best to keep away from them, so I do.

A few girls reject the whole idea of marriage:

> My friends all want to get married soon after they leave school. They can't understand me. It's the last thing I want. I'd like to meet a lot of people. I want to go to other countries and do a lot of maturing.

The pressure to have a boyfriend is the basis of acceptability in your peer group. There is some evidence that Asian girls are less caught up in pressures to 'find a boyfriend', which is often undertaken by the family. This may be one reason why Asian girls actually do better than white girls at school. This is a short-term reprieve, however, as the restriction on their freedom of marriage interferes with their future plans – particularly for higher education: 'Once an Asian girl has finished school, whether she is Hindu, Muslim or Sikh, the threat or prospect of marriage begins to brim over her, casting a blight over her chances of further education – or of a worthwhile working career' (Wilson 1978:100).

Girls who fail to comply with the norms are considered by both girls and boys to be at fault. But a girl faces a situation in which she cannot win. Girls and boys conspire together to ensure that female sexuality is kept strictly under control while male sexuality is given a free rein. As McRobbie and Garber (1976) note, boys who had, sexually and socially, 'sown their wild oats' could 'turn over a new leaf' and 'settle down'; for a girl the consequences of getting known in the neighbourhood as one of the 'wild oats' to be 'sown' was drastic and irreversible.

Girls still talk of the constant fear of being regarded as a tart or a slag, and living alone is seen as too frightening for many girls. The need for protection emerged in a number of the interviews. Charlotte describes how her brother is treated differently from her:

> Boys are a totally different physique. I could go out and be raped whereas he couldn't. He'd have more chance of protecting himself. I think that comes up the whole time. It's not that a boy is more trusted. It's that he's freer.

The harsh reality of existing in a male-dominated world is that you need protection from sexual harassment. Sometimes fathers put restrictions on girls because they are affected by cases of rape in the newspapers and by stories from blokes at work.

Girls can never go out on their own – or even with girlfriends – without fear, though boyfriends are not necessarily any safer. Girls still feel safer with a boy they know:

> Say you have a boy protecting you. It's as if no one can hurt you or nothing. You're protected and everything. If someone does something to you, then there's him there too and it just makes you feel secure.

The threat of male physical violence, as we shall see in Chapter 6, takes its place alongside the verbal abuse to steer girls into the acceptability of a long-term relationship.

Yet a few girls realize that it might be their boyfriend or husband who will assault them. Bridget describes the man she wants to marry as 'someone who will not beat [her] up'.

Not only is it the constraints on an independent sex life that lead girls to marriage, but the family is seen as the 'only hope we appear to have for the fulfilment of needs for warmth and intimacy and love'. Lesbian relationships can offer these, but only if the girl manages to face the pressure towards conformity.

In the face of these strong pressures most girls inevitably subscribe to the idea that they will get married. Nevertheless, their realism leads them to devise ways of rationalizing or

cushioning its inevitable impact. We found four main themes
by which the girls rationalized away the contradiction: by
seeing marriage as inevitable, by delaying marriage, by attributing marriage failure to the wrong choice of partner, and by
seeing marriage as necessary only for the sake of children.

The most important reason girls put forward for marriage is
that they see no realistic alternative. The choice of getting
married becomes a negative one – of avoiding being left on
the shelf. This they see as both a stigma and a danger – there
are risks involved in the life of a single unattached woman:

> If you don't want to get married and want to live a free
> life and you go out with one bloke one week and another
> the next, everyone will call you a tart. Like you've got
> to go out with a bloke for a really long time and then
> marry him.

And there is also the fear of loneliness:

> I'm scared to sleep alone. I'm scared of the dark. I
> wouldn't like to live with my family all my life, but I
> wouldn't like to live alone either.

The fear of being alone is also linked to the question of
security and protection in a male-dominated world, with the
ever-present fear of violence and sexual harassment against
women:

> A boy can go out and just enjoy himself, but a girl can't
> really. She's got to worry. A girl could go out and be
> raped but he couldn't.

Girls can never go out on their own without fear, without
wondering how they will get home at night, without being
careful. Boys too may be at risk of violence on the streets, but
not in the home. Girls are at risk both on and off the streets.
The idea that when a girl gets married she is exercising free
choice fails to take into account these constraints. Alongside
this feeling of physical security in marriage there is the moral
security of respectability. The double standard of sexual morality makes it difficult for a girl to experience any kind of
independent sexual life without being labelled a slag or whore.

When a girl does get a reputation as a slag, all the girls agree that she can only redeem herself by going steady or better still by getting married.

Delaying Marriage

The inevitability of marriage is cushioned for some through a desire to put it off, usually for about ten years. At fifteen, ten years is a lifetime away. As Margaret puts it:

> I don't think about the future at all until it happens. I don't think, 'Oh, what am I going to do in ten years' time?' for a start. I never think that. I think, 'What am I going to do tomorrow?'

By delaying marriage many girls think that they will be able to have some fun, often having fantasies of travel and seeing the world. Michaela explains how marriage is something you end up with after you have 'lived':

> I don't really want to get married 'cos I want to go round the world first like me dad did . . . They got married when they were thirty years old, they just sort of had their life first and then they got married and had us but when you're an air hostess you don't start the job until you're twenty so I want to work until I'm thirty-five.

Boyfriends and marriage can easily interfere with career intentions, and girls can see what has happened to their mums and how little autonomy they have. Some would like to delay marriage in order to develop a career.

> I want to get a start in a good career or whatever, I want to live, have a nice fulfilling life before I actually settle down.

Some girls specifically mention careers:

> I get worried, very worried about my career. You know I need a job . . . My sister ended up in the British Home Stores and she wanted to be a designer. I don't want to end up like her, no way. I just want a decent job.
>
> Q *So you are worried about your future?*

Yes, very worried, I might end up on the streets. How
am I going to support myself if I have a child?

Q *What do you think about getting married?*

My boyfriend were talking about it yesterday. I told him
I wanted to get a job, probably get a car. Then I'd think
about it.

Middle-class girls are often quite clear that they do not
want to be housewives:

If you marry it's not just the man who goes out to work
... I would want to go out too. I wouldn't want to be
stuck in the house because then that's just like a woman's
job, really being stuck in the house and I would want to
go out. I wouldn't like him supporting me. I would want
to stand on my own two feet. Because say he wasn't
there, you'd have to still go out and look for a job.

Many girls realize that the conflict between preparing themselves for a career, boyfriends and marriage can interfere with
a girl's freedom in all sorts of ways. Jasmin, when asked if she
worries whether or not she has a boyfriend, replies:

No. God, they bloody rule your life. When they're there
you don't really want one, but when all your friends
have got one you feel you should have one. I don't really
care if I have one or not.

The conflict between careers and marriage emerges very
clearly from Holland and Eisenhart's (1990) research, where
women who did not get caught up in romantic relationships
did so by postponing or limiting their involvement in various
ways. Some claimed absentee boyfriends who seldom if ever
showed up. One woman gloried in a boyfriend who had a lot
of work and so only had limited time to see her; another
participated diligently in 'man-hunting' activities but when
interviewed never showed any interest at all in finding a
romantic relationship; still others tried to postpone their wed-
ding dates as long as possible and one 'broke up' with the
man she actually intended to marry later.

Women were faced with two dilemmas: how to save face in

what Holland and Eisenhart call the 'sexual auction block', and how to limit their involvement in romantic attachments. They could not avoid being judged mainly in terms of their attractiveness even by professors. Some women saw this as a matter of choice but others saw that women were always vulnerable to being treated from the perspective of sex gender relations.

Choice of Partner

Another way girls avoid the predicament of marriage is to attribute the unhappiness that they see in marriages around them to the wrong choice of partner. The subordinate position that many women find themselves in is often attributed to the lack of good sense in choosing the right husband rather than to the general structural constraints on women at home with young children or on the inequality of sex gender relations. Alice, looking at the 'mistakes' her mother made — in choosing the wrong man — believes:

> But not all marriages are like that, though, are they? Like, if your mum's goes bad, yours might go good. It's what husband you pick.

Alice is right in one respect. Some men allow women more autonomy than others. She does not however criticize the unfairness of the marriage deal itself, particularly if children are involved. Although having children is something most girls want, again, the way in which this inevitably constrains freedom is recognized:

> I think that once you decide to have kids then you are gonna be tied down for a while. That's why it's important not to get married too early — until you're twenty-eight or so.

Romanticism about choosing the 'right man' can be seen as a way of ignoring structural inequalities. Sharon says:

> I would hate to rely on a husband. I see how my mum depends on my dad and it's turned her against him. I'm not going to marry a husband like my mum did. My

dad, he doesn't help at all. I don't see what they see in each other. They must love each other.

But even though she states the contradiction between her mum's grim life and the assumed love between her parents, this does not lead her to question the ideal of 'true love' and look realistically at the material realities of her mum's life. Instead the assumption is that any disadvantages can be avoided by being careful about whom you marry. Annie has made up her mind about whom to avoid:

> I will get someone who doesn't like drinking a lot and just has a little Coke or something.

Several girls mentioned the importance of marrying into a racial group that was acceptable to your parents. Rona, a Greek girl, says:

> My mum lets me go out with boys, but not some, she doesn't mind English or Italian. Never Turkish, God help me. No.
>
> Q *Is this because of religion?*
>
> I think so. They're Muslims and I'm Orthodox and they don't believe in it – and because of the 1974 war. She's happier when my boyfriend is Greek. I could go out with an English boy but I would like him to be really classy . . . I'd prefer him to be Greek.

Though marriage is regarded by most girls as essential for the upbringing of children, cohabitation is increasingly acceptable:

> Actual marriage, I don't think it's necessary unless you're going to have children and I can't visualize myself having children. Apart from that, I don't think actual marriage, a piece of paper, is all that important. I'm not religious or anything.
>
> There are more people living together than getting married. It's all the fashion now.

Living with someone before marriage has the added advantage for Nicky of making divorce unnecessary if the relationship does not work out:

> I think it's better if you live with someone to get to know him better – you don't have to worry about going through a divorce.

Though little research has focused on why boys want to get married, it is apparent that marriage offers material advantages without the restrictions on freedom and financial dependency that women experience. Mira explains how easily a girl can lose self-confidence if she is stuck at home with her married partner going out on the town:

> I think that once you get married you lose pride in yourself, really.
>
> Q *What about boys? Do they lose pride in themselves?*
>
> The ones I know, they don't really lose pride because they sort of go out. They don't have to wear a ring or anything, do they? They still go around free as though they weren't married.

Jessie Barnard (1973) wryly comments: There are two marriages in every marital union, his and hers, and his is better than hers . . . It is men who thrive on marriage. Despite all the jokes about marriage in which men indulge, all the complaints they lodge against it, it is one of the greatest boons of their sex.

In short, the girls are not aware of any positive attraction in married life, yet as far as they see it, once children are on the way, there is not much alternative. Sandy sums it up:

> This idea of love and marriage. I think you're all broken down into thinking you're eventually gonna get married and have kids. If you're really ugly or in a right state or something, then you're not going to – you're not going to go out and meet a bloke. It's like that.

For the Sake of the Children

For many girls having children is the linchpin of marriage. Some middle-class girls reject marriage unless it involves children:

> Actual marriage, I don't think it's necessary unless you're going to have children and I can't visualize myself having

children. Apart from that, I don't think actual marriage, a piece of paper, is all that important. I'm not religious or anything. Living in sin will do me.

Marriage I think of as with children but living together it's different, it's just two people. If you don't want to have children it's OK to live with somebody but if you are going to have children it's better to have a stable family background. So I'd get married if I wanted children.

The idea that having children involves total sacrifice and giving up one's own life comes across constantly:

Children, I'd like them, but not for a long time. Not really until I've sort of lived my life. With children you've got to stay in and you can't go out. You've got to be there all the time.

Girls still see sex roles as rigidly segregated, and looking after children is regarded as naturally the mother's responsibility.

I think men should go out to work because they earn more money than women do. Half the jobs men can do, women can't.

Girls disagreed about how much involvement they wanted from fathers. Many girls welcomed the idea of looking after a baby and did not want any help. They saw children as a means by which they could gain status and influence and did not want any interference. Fran when asked whether she would like to look after a baby replied:

Oh, it'll be lovely. I'd really love it.

Q *Would you expect your husband to help?*

No way. I wouldn't even let him come shopping with me, never mind about help with the baby. I'd like to do it myself. Let him think I'd brought him up with my own hands.

Charlotte, a middle-class girl, strongly disagreed:

I'd get my husband to do half of everything. I don't think it'd be easy but I'd train him. I just don't think it's right that the woman is there to do everything for him.

Marriage is on the whole regarded as necessary for children, but some girls do not take marriage for granted:

> I'd like to marry, say about twenty-eight or thirty, more that age, when you have enjoyed yourself and settled down and have a family. I would want to have a child some time, but not for a long time.
>
> Q *Would that involve marriage?*
>
> It depends. Sometimes I don't see the need for marriage. Maybe it's for the child basically, marriage.
>
> Sometimes it's security sharing a bank account, sort of like that. I don't really see what difference marriage makes.

Some girls regard having children as marking 'the end of your life':

> Children – I'd like them, but not for a long time. Not really until I've sort of lived my life. With children you've got to stay in and you can't go out much. You've got to be there to look after them. You're responsible for someone else.
>
> I certainly want to have kids. I want to be about thirty when I have them. I want to be free from ties until then. I think by the time you're thirty you do want something to hold you down a bit, stop you flying around the place, which I want to do as well.
>
> I think that once you decide to have kids then you've got to accept the fact that you are gonna be tied down for a while. That's why it's important not to get married too early – until you're twenty-eight or so. Just enjoy life when you leave school, leave college.

Some light is thrown on the contradictory way adolescent girls construct motherhood in an article by Prendergast and Prout (1980) based on interviews with fifteen-year-olds about what they thought life was like for mothers at home with young children. On the one hand girls' experience of motherhood in the nuclear family was realistic and unromantic, yet on the other hand they still clung to a sentimental romantic ideology of the joys of motherhood. They found that most of the girls' accounts were dominated by the negative aspects of motherhood – for example, isolation, boredom, and depression. This knowledge seemed to come from girls' observations and judgements and sometimes from their direct experience of childcare. They frequently described their mothers as depressed, but seemed to accept this as something normal and to be expected if you were a mother. Yet the authors found a 'startling change in direction of response between talking of their own mothers and mothers in general: many girls who had given very negative descriptions [of their mothers' experiences at home] went on to agree that in fact life was good for mothers at home with young children'. They made comments like: 'Most women get pleasure in looking after a child. Got someone to look after. Most women have a mothering instinct and want to look after people.' What seemed to count was not their own experience but how mothers ought to feel and behave. The authors argue that:

It can be seen that when children switch from the specificity of their own experience into that of 'mothers' a space is created around their own experiences. Filling this space is what we would call stereotypical knowledge ... Their own experience did not count as knowledge in this respect ... What did count as knowledge was that which is widely available – how mothers ought to feel and behave.

The latter knowledge comes to carry the legitimacy of naturalness which, by denying the former knowledge, effectively prevents a recognition of consequent questioning of any opposition between the two. The researchers point out that the girls' descriptions parallel the themes in Ann Oakley's study of mothers and post-natal depression (Oakley 1981). In her study, most mothers said the whole process – the pregnancy, birth, relationship of mother and child, work of childcare and social position of the mother was different from what they had expected. Four out of five said their expectations had been too 'romantic', 82 per cent said pregnancy was different from what they had envisaged, and motherhood was described by 91 per cent as contradictory to previously held images. These mothers interpreted their inability to cope and live up to the ideal as a failure to be a 'proper mother' and therefore as unnatural. This 'naturalness' of the mother's role acts to deflect concern from the burdens of childcare.

As Prendergast and Prout (1984) suggest, the ways that girls cope with the discrepancy between these two types of knowledge – the normative and the illegitimate – based on their own experience, has much in common with the ways I have suggested girls reconcile the discrepancy between their knowledge of marriage and the universal expectation that that was their natural destiny.

This is however to take an undynamic view and to under-estimate the potential for change in normative views. Girls who are now entering education on far more equal terms than their mothers did, in a very different social climate where feminism is at least on the agenda, and many of whom have seen their mothers struggle with caring for children, often alone and working part-time, may well have a different, less romantic 'normative' view than their mothers who at adolescence had fewer alternative possibilities and certainly were living at a time when equality was not common parlance. This perhaps explains why girls push the idea of the anticipated birth of a child as far away as possible. Every girl I spoke to except one, who wanted to have a large family as early as possible, postponed the whole question of children. They attributed the loneliness to being tied down and knew that motherhood involved sacrificing their independence.

> It depends on the age of the mother. Older mothers are better able to cope. They're more mature. Young ones want to get about, to be free and not held down. I'd get frustrated because it's hard if you are young.

The question of shared childcare rarely arose spontaneously. Sylvia, a middle-class sixteen-year-old, has definite views on this. When asked who would look after the children, she says it should be 'fifty-fifty':

> I think that whoever I'm with – a boyfriend or a husband – whoever it is has got to do half of it as well. It doesn't make any difference if you're a man or a woman. You both should help in that.

Most girls assume that they will take the lion's share, as this is women's role in life.

Boyfriends

Since girls tend to look on any relationship with a boy with marriage in mind, courtship can be seen as a rehearsal for marital life. Often the connection between now and the future is quite explicit:

> The boys are sort of stereotyped men. They'd go off for evenings without the girls and go down to the pub and wouldn't expect the girls to come.

Marcia, a black girl, is quite explicit in her description of boys who 'brag' and Lou, also black, knows which boys to avoid:

> Casanovas, they've got really big heads. They're always going on about the size of their cocks, how big it is, that's the honest truth. They're always on about how big it is. Well that's what Charlie is like.

> The sort of boys I don't like see girls as real conquests, and brag to their friends. You get boys that are flash, they really act big, they think they're it.

Bossiness was often mentioned by Astrid, a white girl, and Mira, an Asian girl:

> Boys quite often don't say what are we going to do, they sort of tell you.

> He's always got to be right, all the time. I'm never allowed to be right, if I know about something and he doesn't. He's always got to be right.

Or taking girls for granted:

A boy that swears and thinks you're easy to please or he just goes round with many girls at a time.

Yeh, he goes, 'Oh, that's my bird, that's my bird,' and then you think you're wanted. You think he loves you and then when you find out he's with someone else he says, 'Oh, what's the matter with you?' Like this, all the time and he really makes you feel as if you're going out with a real big head.

Or treating girls as objects:

It's just the leers blokes give you. The leering sort of look. You know they make you feel like an object for a bloke to look at and touch . . . Just for their satisfaction.

Or being possessive:

People think that it is a girl who wants to get tied down and married but it isn't true. Boys can be really possessive. The ones I go with do, and you have to only go out with them and you can't go out with your friends 'cos a boy might see you and then ask you out and you might like him better. I just have to be free. When you're fifteen you don't really want to get tied down or anything. But you just want to have somebody that you can feel really close to but not act as if you're married, 'cos if you've got somebody they say, 'No, you can't do that.' It's like you're a married couple or something and you're still sort of young and living your life, experiencing everything.

Hitting girls about a bit is accepted by some as natural:

We used to talk about everything really. Just everything you talk to a mate about you could say to him . . . I knew him inside-out really. Every trick like y'know. He used to hit me and that – a bit of a sock, but I still used to like him.

The picture girls give of boys is not clear-cut. Several girls mention that they are attracted to boys they do not particularly like and several complain about 'sloppy boys':

Lots of girls find if you're going out with a bloke you

like, he'll really treat you terrible but you'll like him
more and the ones who treat you all nice and come on
all sloppy about how much they love you, you really
hate them. I've been in the situation where he's been
saying how much he wants to marry me and it really
makes me – ugh. It repulses me. One bloke I really liked
he'd say he'd phone up and he'd never phone, I'd like
him more for that. It's an attraction for girls if someone
can't be tied down. He sort of really plays the Casanova.
Everyone thinks, 'Oh, I'll have a go. I'll try him and
tame him.'

Thus girls are both attracted and repelled by some boys,
but are aware that some boys are chauvinistic and even
violent. The girls themselves are not without ambiguities in
their responses to this, but the overall effect is of the normality
of chauvinism.

Nice boys treat girls as friends who you can 'talk to' and
'trust' (although several girls seem to think it is hard to be
sure you can trust anybody). Age and intelligence are quite
frequently mentioned:

I like them to be old – not old men but sort of nineteen or so.

But more often trust and the way boys treat girls are the
most important criteria – predictably in view of the way boys
customarily treat girls:

I would like to be treated as just equal. I would like to
treat boys the same way as I treat girls – and I like them
to treat me the same as well.

Some girls explain how exciting it is to meet a boy who is fun
to be with but appear surprised if they can talk to him:

He's really exciting to be with. He's so funny. He's got a
really good sense of humour. Sometimes he can act like a
little kid, like, messing about, but then he's all right to
be with . . . You can talk to him . . . I didn't expect to be
able to talk to him as good as I do. I talk to him quite
freely. You do get people who can't really talk to their
husbands or their boyfriends.

Others are not so sure whether they want a boyfriend:

> I don't even care, I don't even know if I want one ... I
> think boys are all the same in some sense. Men think
> girls ought to be quiet. When a girl is with a boy she
> might act tough and a boy thinks she's got to act all soft
> and pathetic.

None the less the normality of chauvinism and non-communication on the part of boys is striking. In spite of this the issue of marriage is still seen by girls as a question of finding a nice boy, scarce as they appear to be. Violence came up in a very matter-of-fact way a number of times, as we shall see in Chapter 6:

> If they're kind and they chat all right and they're just
> kind to you ... If he doesn't go round hitting you and
> punching you as some boys do nowadays ... Say if he
> asks you out and you don't want to go with him, he slaps
> you or something. I don't think that's right.

Hardly an over-romantic view of who to look out for. And the boy to avoid – a Dirty Harry:

> A boy who thinks he can touch up all the girls in the
> world and won't get himself into trouble and when he
> gets one pregnant he hides his face all the time.

Several girls think it was from their fathers that many of the boys' attributes derived. As Mandy comments:

> I think boys get a lot of their attitudes from their dads –
> you know if the dad comes home drunk and he beats up
> his wife the bloke thinks that is how life should be and he
> should go out and get drunk and beat up his girlfriend. I
> don't want to end up like my mum. I'll try and learn
> from the mistakes my mum has made.

Boys and Marriage

Boys, as we have seen, when asked about the future rarely mention marriage. However, most of them see marriage as inevitable. Toby considers it to be a long way off:

> When I'm older I sort of think I should get married so there's someone to keep me company basically, when I get old ... I'd live with the person first rather than just run into it. I don't think about it at the moment. Basically I want a good education.

Their views of marriage are by no means all traditional, some of them even expressing preference for virgins, attractiveness and subservience, but others were more liberal. Bob, when asked in a group discussion what kind of a woman he would like to marry, replied:

> Pretty woman with nice legs, nice tits, nice shoulders, nice face, nice clothes.

A group of Muslim boys I interviewed from Bangladesh and Pakistan were not at all integrated with the white boys in the class. Unlike the white boys' families, half of whose parents were split up, all these boys were from intact homes and none of their mothers worked. They did not contemplate marrying out of their religious group. And their views of women were more traditional than the white boys'. Rajam and Agad, who came to this country when they were six and seven, discuss the kind of girl they would like to marry:

> RAJAM I don't want a girl who will leave you with the washing.
>
> AGAD Not one who starts arguing that she doesn't want to do the housework and she doesn't want to care for the child.
>
> RAJAM I want a girl that is nice, gentle and never has contact with boys.

Imtiaz was critical of girls who did not take a subservient role. When asked what kinds of girls he did not like he answered:

> Girls who don't listen. Girls who want it their own way.
>
> Q *What is wanting it their own way?*
>
> She'll want you to buy this, and buy that. She'd leave you with the washing. They want to control a man.
>
> Q *What kind of control?*
>
> Everything. She'd start arguing. Housework. She'd want

you to take care of the child. I think women should do most of the work in the home.

They were well aware that the world around them was changing. When I asked whether they thought their future wives would work, Rajam replied:

Maybe. Because this is one of the ways that Britain has changed in the last twenty years. Many more women work. They get better grades than the boys. More women are getting jobs as secretaries and part-time. It's not as if they're going to get proper jobs because being a secretary is like freedom in chains.

They predicted divorce spreading to their community:

AGAD The newer generation gets more split up. Most of them do.

Bob, a working-class sixteen-year-old, when asked what kind of girl he would like to marry, wanted a girl who was:

Attractive, clever, nice personality, trustworthy, older, not someone that everyone knows. Not someone who's been out with people I know.

In some interviews boys talked more about the qualities of girls and the importance of 'making her laugh'. All the boys in one group discussion agreed that in their school girls wanted to be like men.

Tomboys. They want to dress like men. Talk like men. Act like men.

Several boys were wary of marriage:

If you get married and you get another girlfriend, you lose money on the divorce.

Marriage costs money. It's stupid getting married as it costs too much.

John thinks it is a good idea as

You can get someone to do your washing and cooking. Though my dad said yesterday, 'Never let a woman in the kitchen.'

The boys' discussion of marriage rarely involved any discussion of relationships. Mike in a group discussion is flippant:

You can't lay a woman in front of the kids.

And Jerry openly declares that violence is useful to keep women in order:

> Women are weaker, so you can get round them by beating them.

A middle-class boy who is anti-racist wants however to avoid feminism:

> I'd never go out with anyone who was a racialist or Women's Lib to a certain extent. It just would get me in such a temper.

Some boys however reject such macho attitudes. When asked whether he would share taking care of children, Tony replies:

> It depends who was bringing home the wage and going out to work. But I'd look on her as an equal. That is the main thing ... I'd want a good relationship, not one where the man goes out to work all day, has his dinner, goes out to the pub and the woman stays in slaving over the kitchen stove all day looking after the kids and not getting a break at all. We'd work out a rota or something, so that both people had a chance to do different things.

Or take this discussion:

> BOY 1 A girl who maybe has good parents. Cause that rubs off [*Laughter*] – no, honestly, it does. A girl you can talk to.
>
> BOY 2 Put it this way, you can get girlfriends just for sex and you can get girlfriends who just wouldn't want to, but it's difficult to find one in between.
>
> Q *You wouldn't have sex if you really liked the girl?*
>
> BOY 2 'Cos I wouldn't, that's the way I am.
>
> BOY 3 So you have certain girls that you like and there are ones who are sex objects? Yeah?
>
> BOY 2 The other day Grace asked me, she said to me, if you've got a girlfriend do I have other girls on the side, and I said, 'No, I don't.' Because if I had a girlfriend I really liked I wouldn't want to hurt her.

BOY 3 Say you go out with a girl and she lets you do what you want and you let her do what she wants. So your relationship don't come into whatever else you do, that's all right.

BOY 2 One boy goes out with one girl, he likes her but he wants something, he wants sex, which he ain't getting. So he goes to the girls he can get it from. So the first girl doesn't like it. Maybe some girls would like it, you never know.

BOY 3 Some boys don't understand girls, it's a code to crack.

For a girl to be keen on sex always carries the risk of being named a slag.

Boys, when asked how they see the advantages of being a boy, are ambivalent about pregnancy, which is seen by some as an advantage and by others as a lack:

Yeah, man, you don't get pregnant.

Some boys complain that men can't have babies, but generally the advantages are unanimously agreed on:

TOM You can stand up for yourself. You can join the army, the navy and the air force. You have more freedom. You can do more things.

JERRY Boys have got the *Sun* newspaper. They've got everything. There's no porno magazines for women. The day you see a porno magazine for women there'd be outrage. In good films you don't see men showing their stuff but with women you do. Men have the power, men have the money. They have everything.

BARRY You can get gay magazines for men.

SAM Everything's for men. So men's sexual desires are catered for by the media. So women don't get exposure to these things at an early age. If a boy opens up the *Sun* there it is.

Q *Do you think that's fair?*

JERRY It's not, but what can you do about it?

SAM That's the way it is. You can't change it.

Boys' views on equality are often contradictory:

> Q *Do you think girls and boys should be equal?*
>
> ZEBHIA Yeah, they should be equal.
>
> Q *Are your mum and dad equal, do you think?*
>
> ZEBHIA Yeah, but my mum never goes out on her own.

A Bengali boy describes how life for his mother is more constricted in this country than abroad:

> ARMAN My mum went out in Bangladesh, our country, but she don't in this country.
>
> Q *How does she feel about that?*
>
> ARMAN She's lonely.
>
> Q *Are there other women around?*
>
> ARMAN Yeah, my aunt's ten minutes' walk from our house. Sometimes I have to take her, to make sure she's safe.
>
> When we come to this country, we're lonely. I've got nobody here. I've only got one cousin, that's it. I want to go back to our country.

Some boys think there are no bad things about being boys, whereas 'girls can't do anything ... unless you are a lesbian' (greeted by gales of laughter). Boys express anxiety about jobs and money and think that girls can always depend on a man to pay for her.

> Girls don't have to worry about money. It's not so important as they can rely on men.

In reality this assumed advantage is debatable. The family can be an even greater source of inequality than the labour market, though that inequality is hidden within the privacy of the domestic economy. Jan Pahl's study (1980) of the distribution of money within the marriage relationship shows how unequal this often is, and other studies indicate that after divorce some women experience a higher standard of living on income support than when they were married, because of their lack of access to the breadwinner's wage during marriage. Overall, of course, women are financially far worse off living alone, when they are usually dependent on the state. This is a situation that concerns the government, which does not want to be burdened with supporting single parents. Carol Smart in her study of marriage breakdown pinpoints the extreme vulnerability of women that is 'hidden much of the time by the structure of the domestic economy, particularly the institution of housekeeping which can masquerade as a wage, or simply by the privacy of domestic life that obscures the extensiveness and special nature of poverty suffered by women' (Smart 1984).

When she asked magistrates in Sheffield whether they thought divorced women on low incomes should be encouraged to work, should receive higher welfare benefits or should receive higher alimony, they disagreed with all such courses of action. Remarriage was seen as the only answer.

The growing number of one-parent families has given rise to alarmist predictions. In 1980 just over one in ten families had one parent. By 1991 this had risen to 15 per cent.[2] Such families have been blamed for everything from the rising crime rate to the decline of civilization. Mary and Michelle of *EastEnders*, the TV soap opera which attracts mass viewing, represented two contrasting pictures of young single motherhood: one mother managed very well, the other, without the help of her family, was buffeted from crisis to crisis.

Girls are seen primarily as potential wives and mothers rather than waged workers. Their identities, their preoccupations and their aspirations are overwhelmingly determined by their common experience of married life, of a future that they now contemplate with a cynicism based on realism and accurate perception, but to which the majority of them, within a few years, reconcile themselves.

Conclusions

What appears to have happened in the last decade or two is that opportunities for women have increased, but little change has occurred in the distribution of responsibility for childcare and domestic work in the home or any recognition by employers of the difficulty of combining work with other responsibilities. In Britain 60 per cent of women with dependent children now work, though predominantly part-time, and in low-paid jobs. According to Cowan, in North America

Men do very little housework . . . Whether men are asked to estimate the time that they spend at housework, or wives are asked to estimate their husband's time or outside observers actually clock the amount of time that men spend at it, no one has ever estimated men's share of housework at anything higher than one and a half hours per day. Housewives who are not employed in the labour market spend, roughly speaking, fifty hours a week doing housework. Housewives who are employed outside the home spend, again roughly speaking, thirty-five hours on their work in and for their homes. Men whose wives are employed spend about ten minutes more a day on housework than men whose wives stay at home (Cowan 1989:20).

Barbara Ehrenreich, writing in 1983 of the American experience, argued that it was men rather than women who were reneging on their family responsibilities and leaving home. According to her argument men had gained 'liberation' and were divorcing and leaving women in dire poverty without the support of a male wage. Although in Britain it appears that more women are leaving men, it is evident that an increasing number of women are living with their children in poverty. In the USA and Britain the dismantling of the Welfare State has made the situation economically far worse for women left with young children. The restructuring of the workforce brought about by the electronic revolution means that many women work part-time, without security, and earn a wage that leaves them below the poverty line. Many women are managing on their own on the breadline, forced into part-time work, often without a male breadwinner to support them and with inadequate nursery and support services. About half of separated men lose contact with their children three years after separation. Women and men would both gain from sharing the responsibility of childcare and moving towards greater equality in marriage. The way masculinity and femininity are constituted in popular discourse is not, in this period of social change, helping them to do so.

In *The Reproduction of Mothering*, Nancy Chodorow (1978) illustrates how socialization processes are gendered. She seeks to explain why it is that women take on a mothering role. She argues that women's responsibility for childcare reproduces particular male and female character structures within the nuclear family of capitalistic society, the female character structure which is characterized by nurturance, dependence and connection and the masculine structure characterized by competitiveness, independence and separation from others. Until our child-rearing practices change and women enter equally into the labour market, the family structure will continue to produce two distinct character structures. There is a discrepancy between these two processes. Women have entered the labour market, but men are not joining them in raising children. Why is this?

Chodorow goes on to argue that since a woman's first relationship (object choice) is her mother, and the transference of love from her mother to a man is not ever complete, women 'remain in a bisexual triangle throughout childhood and into puberty'. They make a sexual resolution in favour of men and their father, but retain an intense emotional triangle and still feel closely connected to their mother and to other women. She suggests that they make this resolution because of taboos against homosexuality and for sound economic reasons. However, because men have such difficulty forming meaningful relationships, their lack of availability and women's less exclusive heterosexual commitment lead women to seek emotional relationships with children, thereby ensuring their mothering. The intense triangle between men and children becomes reproduced. Men, on the other hand, because their first love is their mother, transfer their attachment unambiguously to the woman.

The logic of Chodorow's position is that nothing will change until the domestic and child-rearing systems change. The present system of child-rearing reproduces a character structure that is suited to a particular stage of capitalism but has now become unsuitable as divorce rates and the increase in single-parent households show. The way to break this cycle, which leads to barriers of communication between women and men in later life, is for men to be involved with early child-care. Only by this change will the next generation be able to overcome the unhappiness that women and men are now experiencing. The way masculinity is constituted and reconstituted at adolescence, the most crucial time for identities to develop, is not keeping pace with the economic changes and women's reasonable demands for greater equality. Male identity is still defined negatively by society's denunciation of male participation in female work. The media has a particularly pernicious influence here. Even in the current baby-boom movies (see, for example, *Kramer versus Kramer* and *Three Men and a Baby*) we are presented with an image of men usurping woman's child-rearing rather than joining reciprocally into it.

We are moving towards a society that has a diversity of forms of child-rearing. The consequences of the oppression of women in the family are far-reaching for both sexes. It is not only women who suffer from such a distortion and splitting of human experience. Men, though they may not realize it, in some ways lose out more than women. Often their relationships with their children are tenuous and superficial. Their relationships with other men can be spoiled by competitiveness and ambition, and their relationship to work, where the pursuit of profit reigns more strongly than ever, leads many men to spend little time at home and is a major reason for marriage breakups. The nuclear family prescribes a clear-cut distinction between the sexes and a particular form of relating as appropriate which is no longer adaptive to the changing economy. This should involve both a commitment to looking after children jointly, as well as contributing financially.

In the next chapter I will consider to what extent girls' experience of school prepares them for the dual role as paid worker and wife and mother.

Notes

1. The OPCS 1989 survey showed that the number of weddings in England and Wales dropped in 1989 to 348,000, while divorces rose by 2,000 more than the previous year.

The number of divorces doubled between 1971 and 1982 and now one couple in four can expect their marriage to break up within twenty years and four in ten marriages will end in divorce. For those with children, one child in five will see their parents divorce before reaching the age of sixteen. During the 1980s the divorce rate continued its upward spiral.

2. According to the 1990 General Household Survey, lone parents headed 18 per cent of families with dependent children – children aged under sixteen or sixteen to eighteen if in full-time education and living at home. Between 1987 and 1990 the proportion of families headed by an unmarried mother rose from 4 per cent of all families to 6 per cent, from 5 per cent to 7 per cent by a divorced mother and from 2 per cent to 4 per cent by a separated mother.

Bibliography

Barnard, J., 1973, *The Future of Marriage*, Souvenir Press

Brown, G., and Harris, T., 1978, *The Social Origins of Depression*, Tavistock

Chodorow, N., 1978, *The Reproduction of Mothering: Psychoanalysis and the Sociology of Gender*, University of California Press

Cowan, R. S., 1989, *More Work for Mother*, Free Association Books

Ehrenreich, B., 1983, *The Hearts of Men*, Pluto Press

Family Policy Studies Centre, 1990, *Family Changes*

Greer, G., 1971, *The Female Eunuch*, Paladin

Holland, D., and Eisenhart, M., 1990, *Educated in Romance: Women, Achievement and College Culture*, University of Chicago Press

Jephcott, P., 1942, *Girls Growing Up*, Faber and Faber

Jones, A., 1991, *Women Who Kill* (Foreword by Bea Campbell), Victor Gollancz

Jordan, T., 1990, *Growing Up in the 1950s*, Optima

Kristeva, J., 1989, *Tales of Love*, Columbia University Press

Leonard, D., 1980, *Sex and Generation*, Tavistock

McRobbie, A., 1978, 'Jackie: An Ideology of Adolescent Femininity', Stencilled Occasional Paper No. 53, Women Series, Birmingham CCCS

McRobbie, A., 1981, 'Just Like a Jackie Story', in McRobbie, A., and McCabe, T. (eds.), *Feminism for Girls: An Adventure Story*, Routledge and Kegan Paul

McRobbie, A., 1991, *Feminism and Youth Culture: from 'Jackie' to 'Just Seventeen'*, Macmillan

McRobbie, A., and Garber, J., 1976, 'Girls and Subcultures: An Exploration', in Hall, S., and Jefferson, T. (eds.), *Resistance Through Ritual*, Hutchinson

Modleski, T., 1991, *Feminism Without Women*, Routledge and Kegan Paul

Oakley, A., 1981, *From Here to Maternity*, Penguin

Pahl, J., 1980, 'Patterns of Money Management Within Marriage', *Journal of Social Policy*, 9, No. 3

Prendergast, S., and Prout, A., 1980, 'What will I do . . .? Teenage girls and the Construction of Motherhood', *Sociological Review*, August 1980

Sharpe, S., 1976, *Just Like a Girl*, Penguin

Smart, C., 1984, *The Ties That Bind*, Routledge and Kegan Paul

Stafford, A., 1991, *Trying Work*, Edinburgh University Press

Willis, P., 1977, *Learning to Labour*, Saxon House

Wilson, D., 1978, 'Sexual Codes and Conduct', in Smart, C., and Smart, B. (eds.), *Women, Sexuality and Social Control*, Routledge and Kegan Paul

Chapter 4
Education

My mum she could have gone to university but she got married. It just happens, doesn't it? But I'm more ambitious than she was. I would go mad if I didn't have a career (Moira, aged fifteen)

Working in a corner shop, not taxing your brain – it seems such a waste going to school all this time and then not doing anything worthwhile (Haylee, aged sixteen)

What are girls educated for? In what way are girls' and boys' lives at school different? Are we educating girls to fit into society as it is now, where women do most of the housework and childcare on top of a job, or are we educating them for equality? And if we are educating them for equality, what kind of equality are we talking about?

The education system has recently been fundamentally reformed. The Education Act 1988 requires girls and boys for the first time to be offered the same curriculum. It will no longer be possible for girls to avoid maths and sciences, which they often consider to be 'male' subjects. The Education Act embraces a clear commitment to equal opportunities for girls and boys. But is the model of equal opportunities held by government educationalists appropriate for our rapidly changing society? Is the education we offer boys any longer appropriate? And does equal opportunities just mean educating girls like boys? Now we are moving from a model of progressive education to an education focused more narrowly on work, on competitiveness and individualism, are girls joining boys in an education that relegates emotional and caring qualities to the private sphere and renders those qualities inferior? These are some of the controversial debates which I shall refer to in describing the experience of girls and boys at school.

There are three broadly divergent views of the aims of education for girls: the first sees education as liberating girls from their relegation to the home and the second regards education as a way of reproducing subordination of class, race and gender. In relation to gender, girls receive all sorts of contradictory messages about whether their future lies in marriage (combined perhaps with unskilled, low-paid work) or in careers. These messages entail core dilemmas of their sexual and social identity. The girl who prioritizes a career may face taunts over her lack of femininity and will have to reconcile her career aspirations with her relationship to boys and the pressures towards domesticity and marriage. Girls at school have often been described by teachers as docile and quiet and, if successful, as 'hard workers' rather than clever. The third approach to education emphasizes that girls resist the messages they receive and develop different strategies to pave their way through the educational system. This is an interactionist approach. Four different ways girls deal with the contradictions between schooling and femininity will be discussed. Finally I will discuss what I mean by the feminization of schooling.

Aims of Education

Is education geared towards preparing girls to be wives and mothers, as was historically the case, or is it educating them primarily for employment, overtly denying that they will be combining the roles of homemaker and paid worker? According to the functionalist school of education, the major purpose of education is to prepare girls and boys for their respective roles in society. If members of a group do not do well at work, it is because they do not do well at school. Therefore, if women are unequal in the workforce, then better opportunities should be provided for them at school. In Britain girls now achieve higher qualifications than boys at sixteen and comprise 45 per cent of the labour force. Women who work are on the whole better educated than men, yet their position within it has not improved. Their status and pay are markedly lower than mens, and few women are promoted into positions of power in the professions, the arts, education, politics, the civil service or industry. Women hit what has been called the 'glass ceiling'.[1] Various explanations are offered for why women have made so little progress towards equality at work. One argument attributes the inequality to an organization of work where family responsibilities are consigned to women in the private sphere and these responsibilities take priority over promotion at work. Another argument attributes inequality to discriminatory attitudes and practices of men at all levels of society who oppose women's equality due to the entrenched sexist attitudes they developed during adolescence.

Education for Liberation or for Subordination?

Education can be seen as a way of liberating women or of reinforcing their inferiority, by preparing them for their position in society as wives and mothers. As a goal education has been fought for and seen as a route to equality. Mary Wollstonecraft in 1792 considered education to be the most important pathway to women's liberation. She passionately disagreed with Rousseau, the French philosopher, who proposed that women should be educated to be subservient and pleasing to men. He described the reasoning woman as a monster on the grounds that women would lose their femininity if they developed reasoning powers. Wollstonecraft saw education and the development of reason as the path to liberation for women not to threaten men but to develop their potentialities. 'This is the very point I aim at. I do not wish them to have power over men, but over themselves' (Wollstonecraft 1792). The association between reason and masculinity, and its opposition to emotionality, which is associated with femininity, is a dichotomy that feminists argue has many unfortunate consequences.

The education system in Britain has been fundamentally restructured with the enactment of the 1988 Education Act which introduced a core curriculum to be followed by all girls and boys for the first time. Alongside this, the government is moving away from a progressive form of education to a more overtly functionalist system, geared towards preparing children for employment in a highly competitive capitalist economy. Higher education has been affected by this ethos with the emphasis on 'enterprise'. The paradox is that this is occurring at a time of deep economic recession and rising unemployment.

Education does not of course self-consciously, formally, prepare girls and boys differently. It is not an overt but a latent process. School is supposed to prepare people to come out of the family into the alienating bureaucratic male world – the world of rationality. A distinction has been made between the manifest, the overt aims of education and the latent social function which prepares girls and boys for their position within a hierarchical, classist and racist society. In the case of girls, this 'hidden curriculum' prepares them for marriage and domesticity, and for subordination at work. It even discourages them from challenging the educational ethos, by demanding that they 'keep quiet' and hide their sexual difference.

Sceptics of the value of the educational system have argued that it is designed to reproduce the class system, to prepare most children for subordination through disciplining them and, according to Illich, a progressive educationalist who wrote a book called *Compulsory Miseducation*, by teaching pupils that they are ignorant, that they have no autonomous skills and that the teacher is always right. Therefore education prepares a population for a world over which they are socialized to have no control. Illich is talking about class but the same could be said about gender.

Similarly girls, it could be argued, experience schooling as a preparation for domesticity and subordination to men. Girls are taught that they are inferior to boys. For example, I shall show how girls 'service' boys in the classroom by lending them equipment and that boys 'hog' the equipment such as the table-tennis board, preventing girls from having a turn.

The process that goes on in classrooms does not mean that girls passively accept teachers' or boys' definitions and views of femininity, as we all have ways of making sense of our experience and sometimes reject the messages we receive. This is well documented in the sociology of education. The most sophisticated analysis of this 'interactionist' position comes from Paul Willis's (1977) analysis of working-class boys' resistance to education in *Learning to Labour*. In explaining why working-class lads take on lower-working-class jobs Willis argues that the rejection of school and the development of a counter school culture is a rehearsal for the realities of lower-working-class life. He provides a convincing description of how the lads adopt an aggressive male identity in order to reject liberal pedagogy. The creation of gender identities can only be understood through this interactionist method. One way of applying this type of analysis to girls would be to argue that for girls there are a number of strategies, analogous to but significantly different from that identified by Willis, whereby girls insulate themselves from the career-orienting aspects of education for lives of subordination.

We are talking here about a dynamic process involving conflict and resistance. In this way some girls reject schooling and only gain a sense of identity to the extent to which they rebel. Girls, as we shall see, adopt a range of strategies, from expressing a heightened form of femininity, to 'keeping quiet' or becoming rebels or tomboys. Like the lads, some say 'Why should I swot?' For them the answer to this question is that, at least for working-class girls, they are all likely to end up as mothers and housewives where academic qualifications will be irrelevant. Many girls find being provocative to teachers or having fun with each other is a more 'rational' response to the experience of schooling than concentrating on academic work. So within the education system which claims to be universally fair, just and impersonal is embedded an implicit preparation for girls' domesticity. Even if girls can succeed in their careers, they are succeeding in joining a culture prepared for them by powerful males. For women to succeed is to connive with that which celebrates their subordination.

Studies of girls' educational experiences at school have documented the ways the school contributes to reproducing and sustaining gender inequalities and identities. Researchers (Spender 1982, Deem 1984) have shown how the school works ideologically to prepare girls to accept their role as low-paid workers or unpaid domestic wives and mothers. This literature has shown how during the nineteenth century the education system was structured as much by gender as by class. Girls were educated either for domesticity or to be 'cultured wives'. The post-war development of equality of opportunity initiatives by and large ignored gender: class was the focus. It had long been recognized that a major aim of educational policy should be to try and overcome the disadvantages that children carry with them from their home and class background into an educational system formally committed to equality. Latterly this concern has been extended to cover race. Thus while the influence of class background and factors surrounding race have been recognized as impediments to the equality of opportunity, gender inequalities have not been seen as obstacles at all. As late as 1963 an education system committed to formal equality was seen by the Newsom Report as a weakness from the standpoint of educating girls:

We try to educate girls into becoming imitation men and as a result we are wasting and frustrating their qualities of womanhood at great expense to the community . . . In addition to their needs as individuals our girls should be educated in terms of their main social function – which is to make for themselves, their children and their husbands a secure and comfortable home and to be mothers.

Official government reports until recently accepted the role of women as wives and mothers doing unpaid work in the home and failed to recognize that women also did paid work.

Increasingly, however, with the influx of married women into the workforce, governments have had to recognize women's paid work. In the progressive 1980s, following sex discrimination legislation both in the USA and the UK, equal opportunity policies were put on the agenda. Attempts to break down the gender differentiation of subject choice led Jane Marshall to observe: 'It was concluded that girls could now learn woodwork and boys could become a bit more domesticated. Bright girls could perhaps take sciences, competing alongside boys for high status professions. Boys could relax, take it easy, and at last do some girls' subjects without losing face' (Marshall 1983).

However a broader conceptualization of equality of opportunity has not in practice been easy to achieve. Most initiatives have narrowly focused on issues such as subject choice, no longer so relevant with the introduction of the national curriculum which all pupils, male or female, have to follow. The formal structures of education have changed radically since the last century. It is no longer a question of girls being openly educated for domesticity (as described by Deirdre Beddoe in *Discovering Women's History*, the curricula dealing with needlework, household management, cookery, laundry techniques, etc.). But the educational system cannot be exhaustively described simply in terms of its formal aims and institutional practices surrounding the teaching process. Schools in the USA and Britain, for example, spend far more on boys outside as well as inside the classroom, most particularly on sports programmes. The sexism of the curriculum is nowadays a more subtle process.

The first point to emphasize about the dynamics of sexism is the need to look beyond the formal organization of the school as an institution to the cultural and social interaction that goes on in and around school life. The social and cultural life of the school is not insulated from that of the family and the neighbourhood which surrounds it. School life is an aspect of social life in general. This means that there is strong pressure on girls, regardless of their social class, to regard marriage and domesticity as the main aim of life and their work in the

labour market as secondary. Housework is crucial here and
girls are already spending a significant amount of their school
time undertaking it. Yet recent studies of adolescence (Coleman 1990) do not even mention housework as a relevant
aspect of their lives. This pressure is daily reinforced in social
and family life and will also be reflected in the social life of
the school, exercising an influence far more powerful than
the formal aspects of school organization or the structure of
the curriculum. So when Sandy and Marianne are asked how
they see themselves in five years' time, they reply:

> In five years' time? Right, so I'm twenty-one, right? I see
> myself pushing a pram. I don't see myself working.
> Probably married, a housewife with kids.

When Imtiaz, a fifteen-year-old Bengali boy, is asked the
same question he answers quite differently:

> In five years' time, I hope I'm working and not on the dole.

All the boys I interviewed, except for Ashak, an Asian
fifteen-year-old boy, answered this question in terms of work,
none mentioned marriage and family unless specifically asked.
Ashak, whose father has been unemployed for four years,
when asked this question, said he saw himself dead. His
concern is mainly the fear of unemployment:

> All the people unemployed. People ain't going to have
> jobs. It's bollocks. One day even doctors won't have jobs.

This leads to my second point, that much of what turns
even the formal educational process in a sexist direction is
derived from the social dynamics of the classroom. As far as
girls are concerned this is associated with the classroom behaviour of boys and the response of teachers. The co-ed/single-sex
distinction in British schools is important for girls because
what steers the formal learning process in a sexist direction
often stems from the presence of boys in the classroom, and
their effects on teachers' attention and time devoted to girls,
sexual harassment of girls and the ability of girls to hold their
own in competition with boys. 'We get glimpses of the extent
of boys' disruption of the classroom: their noisiness, their

sexual harassment of girls, their demands for attention and their need of disciplining and their attitudes to girls as the silent or the "faceless" bunch' (Arnot 1984).

Thirdly, many of the girls are already participating in their future roles of domestic labour to the detriment of their schoolwork, by helping mother with housework, sometimes to the tune of fourteen to sixteen hours a week. According to domestic ideology, young women should prioritize family relationships over schoolwork. Schooling ignores the significance of domestic unpaid work. The assumption is that this work is woman's work and certain jobs are unnatural for women because of the difficulties of combining paid and unpaid work. Housework is a constant bone of contention as girls with brothers are often made to clean out their brothers' rooms. Girls are expected and socialized into helping their mothers with domestic tasks. To be forced to undertake domestic tasks rather than their homework carries the message that schooling is not a serious undertaking for girls.[2]

Housework

The amount of time spent on housework is still compatible with McRobbie's finding that fourteen- to sixteen-year-old girls attending a youth club spend between fourteen and sixteen hours a week on domestic work and are not joined in this work by their brothers (McRobbie 1978). Class differences are important too. Isabelle, a middle-class girl, perceptively says:

> It's got to do with your parents, your background, your upbringing. 'Cos if you mix with different people their mums and dads treat school in a completely different way . . .
> Q *Can you give me an example of the difference?*
> I think maybe say if you take a day off school or something, some of their mums like them to take a day off to help them, but my mum wouldn't.

Frequently girls who do domestic work complain that it interferes with their homework, although they seem to think it

reasonable for their mums to ask for some help. The amount
of help varies. Some girls report a heavy load, especially if
their mother is houseproud:

> My mum is very houseproud ... I do three jobs a week
> and dry up every night. Like yesterday I went to the
> baths and done three hours' washing ... Well, at least
> from five p.m. to seven p.m. and I ironed it all for her, I
> did an hour and a half's ironing. Day before, I do out
> the bedroom, cleaned the bath and made my bed. It's
> my mum, she's so clean you can't drop a crumb.

Sheila says she does forty-four hours a week housework:

> On Saturday I spend most of the day – five to six hours
> a day I help my mum and on Sunday I don't go out at
> all. I'm indoors helping to clean up the place, so it's
> about forty-four hours altogether.

And she even takes her mum's paid job:

> It takes me just over an hour at night and I get £1.50 a
> night for it ... It's supposed to be my mum's job but she
> gives it to me. They don't know 'cos I'm too young.

Some girls resent doing their brothers' cleaning:

> My mum tells me to clean out my brothers' bedrooms.
> I've got three brothers, it's their bedroom, why don't they
> clean it? They dirty it, why don't they tidy it? My mum
> says, 'You're a girl, you do it.' So I say, 'I wish I was a boy.
> Just pretend I'm a boy then,' but she still picks on me.

Jacky objects strongly to the double standard:

> I just don't think it's right that the man should think
> that the woman is there to do everything for him.
>
> Q *So does your mum do everything?*
>
> We have to help, me and my brothers, and my brothers do
> as much as I do. So that's good, and he's working as well.

Jacky's experience is unusual. Tania complains that boys
get away with murder:

> Like a girl can work in a bakery, launderette, chip shop or
> anything, but with a boy they don't expect them to go to
> work. My mum just gives him the money and everything.

He's lazy. We all say our brothers are lazy, they don't help
with the housework or anything. But we've got no choice.

The National Child Development Study (Fogelman 1976)
found half the sample of 12,000 sixteen-year-olds surveyed
work in term-time, though the number of hours worked varied.
When this is added to domestic responsibilities it is not negligible. A study of Canadian girls found that 85 per cent are
regularly expected to do household chores and half of them
take a major responsibility for housework for the whole family
(Gaskell 1992). In their descriptions of who did the housework,
it is clear that mothers take most of the responsibility, girls
help most and boys rarely do much. Even young women who
said they didn't do much in fact listed household chores that
they regularly do. They conclude that females' responsibility
for this work is so deeply ingrained that it is barely noticed
(Gaskell 1992: 77).

In my study, the amount of housework girls undertake depends
on parents' attitude to schooling and career. The picture of only
girls participating in domestic work is not completely clear-cut,
and with more women in the labour force it appears to be
changing. Diana Reay (1990) in a recent study of thirty-five boys
at a north London primary school discovered that many of the
boys did at least four to five hours of housework every week. Only
three did none. One boy calculated that he did over twelve hours.
A number looked after baby brothers and sisters. She also found
that her stereotypes of the boys were too simplistic and many of
them showed their feelings when upset, sometimes by crying.

In my interviews with boys some boys claimed they did
housework, though not nearly so much as the girls. Jerry said,
for example,

I always do the washing-up when my dad wants me to.
Sometimes I cook for the whole family, like if we have a
barbecue. My dad taught me everything I know. Everything my mum can make, I can make. I do the Hoovering
and some housework. My sister used to do it but she's gone
now. I never leave it all to my mum, never. I spend about

three to four hours on housework a week. My mum would never let me stay off school to help in the house.

Tony, who wants to be a lorry driver and lives with his mother who is divorced, admits he only helps in the house when he feels like it, which is not very often. He says he occasionally tidies his room and Hoovers, but he never washes his clothes. Sean, on the other hand, who wants to be a cartoonist, says he often helps in the house:

> I help often. Wash up, cook sometimes. I clean up my own room, always clean the bath, vacuum occasionally. But washing-up and cooking are the main jobs I do.

Girls' Different Approaches to School

By stressing the nature of school both as a formal teaching structure and curriculum and as a system of social relations between girls, between girls and boys, and with teachers, we can understand the variety of ways in which the girls in this study talk about school. For example, some girls are pro-school, and like going to school but are very much alienated from the teaching process. By contrast, others want to learn, are strongly oriented towards the formal teaching process but are bored and alienated from school for various reasons. A complete map of the different positions would look like this:

Pro-school

	Pro- learning		Anti- learning
	Academic, career orientated	Pro-school for social rather than learning activities	
	Learning orientated but alienated from school	Little interest in either learning or social activities	

Anti-school

We thus have four groups of girls, or rather four possible strategies that girls could be pursuing towards the school and its role in their lives, and sexism features as a factor in each strategy in a different way.

Academic and Pro-school

> I think school's really nice. It's a really nice atmosphere. The teaching is really good.
>
> I just love school. This school is very free though academically it's very strong. It does give you some freedom as well as achieve good grades. I don't feel pressured.

There is a distinct group of academic and career-oriented girls in the study. They are most likely to be middle-class girls who are minimally aware of their disadvantages by comparison with boys in the learning process. Girls are excelling at gaining formal qualifications. In single-sex girls' schools, their level of achievement is particularly high, higher indeed than boys'. If the dynamics of those disadvantages are in any case associated with the presence of boys – for example, boys attract a disproportionate amount of teachers' time – then of course such disadvantages are minimized in a single-sex school. The attitudes of girls to school in the single-sex school differ from the mixed comprehensive. Girls attending the single-sex school are on the whole far more work-oriented and positive in their approach to teachers than in the other two schools. In many single-sex schools the aim is to improve the position of women, emphasizing intellectual development rather than development of the skills of domesticity and motherhood. The ethos of the school may therefore be every bit as important as whether it is single-sex or mixed. The girls at the single-sex school in my study were more aware of the hazards of marriage:

> I think it's important to do well at school. If you can't get a job, or something . . . Especially nowadays, it's hard to get one.
>
> It's very liberated here but that's just because it's a girls' school. All the teachers are trying to get you out and get

a good career and at another school, at a mixed school I think there's something wrong with you if you don't get out and get a career. They think it's great if you don't want children and you don't want to get married.

Not all teachers appear to be aware of the contradictions girls face. As we have seen in the previous chapter, girls at sixteen do not usually aspire to marriage, which they view realistically, but girls from all social classes generally talk in terms of having a career or at least working outside the home. There is a degree of fantasy in the way girls talk about careers, motivated by escape or postponement of the inevitability of marriage. Being an air hostess, so 'you could travel the world' is often regarded as the height of ambition. The reality of the job, a 'waitress in the sky', is rarely foreseen.

Few of the girls even in this group actually go on to successful careers, and the evidence suggests the drop in any aspirations is rapid. There are of course plenty of girls in all social classes in the mixed comprehensives who want to learn and do want careers. Some fantasize about careers in order to delay thinking about marriage, and it is not until after their school-leaving certificates that girls as a group fall behind boys as they reconcile themselves to the reality of marriage and poor opportunities. But they do not have to do this by developing a subculture in opposition to the school, like Willis's lads, because at school teachers' attitudes, subtle pressures as regards subject choice, parental pressure, poor career opportunities and – in mixed schools – the attitude and behaviour of boys, all combine to push them in this direction. The enthusiasm of such girls for careers at this age is quite striking:

I want to learn more now. I don't just want to work in Woolworth's. I mean, even if I do get my exams I don't want to do something like work in a shop . . . I want to do something that I like doing.

I think I'm just as capable, or more capable than a lot of boys. I know I could get a good job and it annoys me when they start immediately presuming just because you're a girl, you know, they're going to be the ones who go out and you're going to be the ones to stay at home, even if you're more intelligent than them.

Irene Payne (1980) in describing the experience of being educated in a single-sex girls' school describes how the school had an 'official' attitude to boyfriends, which was that 'girls did not have time for them'. Payne suggests this was one way of denying sexuality, but surely there is also some truth in the view that for girls to deal with all the implications of what having boyfriends involves in regard to their sexual reputation, quite apart from the ups and downs of sexual relationships, means there is some point to such a policy.

Academic but Anti-school

Irrespective of class, many girls in mixed schools want to learn and have careers but are alienated from school. This appears to be particularly true of West Indian girls in British schools. One study, for example, found that West Indian girls conformed to the notion of the 'good pupil' by working hard, but behaved badly in class and were anti-school. Being pro-learning and pro-school do not necessarily go together (Fuller 1980). Mirza (1992) in a larger study found a similar picture in two schools in the Midlands, where black girls did rather better than boys, both black and white, but did not conform to the school culture. Grace Evans (1980) one of the first black women teachers to write about her experiences, came to similar conclusions. A common complaint of white teachers was to talk about black girls as 'loud' and confrontational, threatening the authority of the teacher. She explains how the price of a good education, a European education in short, was and still is the denial of one's black cultural identity:

The price of a good education was attained at the cost of great sacrifice on the part of one's parents, sometimes the whole family. Aside from this cost, another price is paid by the recipient of an education, and this is the personal cost of the process of de-culturalization, or de-Africanization, whereby all personal expressions of one's

original African culture are eliminated and European codes established instead ... It includes training the body to adopt European
body language and gesture, and the voice to adopt European tones
of speech and non-verbal expression. Loudness is discouraged, as it
reflects field life and rural peasant status.

Teachers share attitudes about what is appropriate feminine
behaviour, which can affect their assessments of girls. Speaking
in an unfeminine way can categorize you not only as a
slag but also as unintelligent. The interrelationship of classist,
racist and sexist assumptions about children is complex.
Marcia, a black girl, says:

> It's who she likes. If you are a big-mouth who likes to
> back-chat her, she chucks you in the CSE group and if
> you're a softy, you know, listen and don't talk a lot, she
> puts you in the O-level.

Research indicates that a significant proportion of teachers
are racist and many show little understanding of other cultures
(see Brah and Minhas 1985, Mirza 1992). Black girls in my
research complained that teachers underestimated their ability:

> I want to go in for pharmacy, but they [the teachers]
> said it's a man's job.

Isatou, an Asian girl, speaks of her career-advisory teacher
in the following way:

> She puts everybody off. She's another one prejudiced
> isn't she? She seems like she wants you to end up in
> Tesco's packing beans.

Increasingly, recent research findings have challenged the
notion that black children necessarily have a poor self-concept
resulting from racism and sexism in the school (see Stone
1985). Amrit Wilson makes a distinction between black children under and over twelve in her study of Asian schoolgirls.
The younger ones are too young to fight racism and it is as
though they are stunned into accepting the inferiority with
which white society has labelled them. But at twelve their
feelings seem to change and their inferiority clears away
(Wilson 1978:93). She describes girls attacking girls in Harles-

den. Sharma, aged twelve, says, 'They call you Pakis, things like that and if you answer back you are really in serious trouble. Then they get their friends to beat you up' (1978:96).

Some look on the opportunity to mix with girls and boys from different cultural backgrounds very positively. Mark, for example, says:

> I think the only way you can get a good multi-cultural education is being in a school with lots of different cultures. I mean, you can't learn this sort of thing in an all-English school or a Catholic school, you can't learn about Asian religions or whatever. I find religion very interesting.

Racism, of course, involves more than interpersonal stereotypes, which we have discussed in Chapter 1. The relations between girls are not the only terrain on which the massive institutional racism of British society makes its impact. Treatment by police, the denial of job opportunities, treatment by teachers lie alongside the relationships between the girls. Several girls mentioned their parents' and teachers' racism:

> My dad's quite a racialist. My mum and I have worked on him a bit. But I won't discuss it with him. I get very embarrassed. He sort of says all these things about all black people commit crimes and there was me and one other girl who were prepared to stand up to him in a group of eight. All the others were having a go. I really belittled him in front of everyone. He got me so angry that I couldn't help it.
>
> Q *Do you get much racism in school?*
>
> Not really. Girls don't show a lot really but the teachers are.

The common assumption made by some researchers that black girls' self-concept would be damaged by the experience of racism has not been supported by the few studies of adolescent black girls that have been undertaken. This may be due to the more dominant position of women in Afro-Caribbean families. Black Afro-Caribbean women are more likely than white women to be working full-time and are more often single parents. Though this undoubtedly puts great pressure on them and means they are more likely to suffer from low income and all its concomitants, the mothers may provide a strong role-model for their daughters. Ann Phoenix (1987) points out in her research that in the intact family, the low status ascribed to black men in British society means that power in the family may not be distributed in the same way as in an intact white family. Rather than viewing black women as doubly oppressed, it may be that their position is different but not necessarily inferior to the position of black men who both in the public sphere and the private sphere are marginalized. In one study of girls of Afro-Caribbean origin in a south London school, girls did not see themselves as future dependants and intended to pursue diverse careers, though they were not unaware that they might land up in jobs traditionally done by women. There is also evidence that Asian and Afro-Caribbean girls tend to be more critical of the mythical ideal of romantic love and marriage than their white peers (see Griffin 1985), and to be more committed to educational success.

Holland and Eisenhart's study of campus life in the USA also found differences between black and white girls in their approach to learning. The black girls were concerned not so much with 'doing well' as 'getting over', i.e. gaining a qualification. According to American studies (Fordham and Ogbu 1986), black students are torn between an individualistic ethos encouraged by school officials and a collectivist ethos promoted by peers. For some black students, doing well at school is equated with 'selling out' or becoming non-black. 'The burden of acting white was too high a price to pay for academic success' (Ward 1990).

Another reason for many girls' alienation from school is the presence of large numbers of other girls who have already abandoned the orientation to career and work:

> There are only three in the class who want to work. We can't work properly though, 'cos they just mess around and we try to do some work but then they just come up to us and make a lot of noise so that you can't work. One

day the teacher was trying to teach us and they suddenly come into the classroom. They started crowding around our desks singing, stuff like that, being really stupid. You can't go and tell the teacher and tell on them 'cos then they start picking on you even more and saying that you need a teacher to help you and all that. Even if you tell them to shut up, they start on you even more.

Pro-school, Anti-work

That's the one good thing about school, friends.

It's not work I like. School is just a place for meeting my friends and having a laugh.

Sometimes I'm depressed and I think, 'Why should I bother going to school?' If it wasn't for your friends you wouldn't go . . . Some of the teachers are like robots. Nothing goes in.

Some girls are not interested in work but still value school life as a form of contact with friends. As Janey says:

What makes school fun is seeing your mates.

Not all girls were keen on the view of school as a centre for social life. Dorrie is disparaging about such girls:

They just like mucking around. They don't want to work. They don't play table-tennis. They just sit around talking about boys, most of the time doing nothing. They're show-offs. They just muck around the streets causing trouble. They muck around with your books and start drawing all over you with chalk. They start throwing around your books and there's nothing you can do about it. They exaggerate. They say, 'I went out last night.' If they had to get in by ten, they say it was twelve. If you say anything they hit you.

And Kate adds:

School. I know I have to come and it's good for me. I want to learn and get a good job but I don't like working. I find it boring. We throw things at each other or shout all the time or argue. It makes school life a bit less boring. You say, 'Oh I'm going to work,' then it's the same thing all over again you get bored.

Many of the girls in this category find school boring, irrelevant and involving constant conflicts. Girls who come to school for mainly social reasons are often thwarted by teachers who continually try to harass them into working. Teachers do not seem to be very successful in this task. Some girls develop very antagonistic relationships with them, but other teachers appear to have either given up on them or to treat them more sympathetically, particularly if they keep quiet. Take Maureen's view:

> There're a lot of groups that are work oriented. I'm in the same group as my friends because I suppose we're the same sort of ability. And all the others are the same as their friends. You're more influenced by your friends, like to work or not to work, then you're gonna be in the same group as them ... I'm pretty lazy, I just can't be bothered to do it. I think it's because I don't like studying and they don't press me now.

Leah on the other hand complains that:

> I enjoy school, but when you want to chat you just can't. You want to talk all the time and you have to listen. It gets on my nerves and it gets on the teacher's nerves because they think you're being rude. You are, but you're not meaning to, you just want to talk. You don't get enough breaks so you want to chat.

Girls often put forward a number of reasons why it is not worth concentrating on academic work. These range from the expectation that work for them will be part-time, something they fit in with their family responsibilities, to girls who think appearance is more crucial than qualifications. The way that women's bodies are often involved in the deal between women workers and their employers (see Cockburn 1991) is a concern to many girls. Gita, an Asian girl, sees attractiveness as vital for a successful career, and is more worried about that than about her schoolwork:

> I wish I had a nice figure, especially for my career. I wish I had a better body. I think I'm too skinny.

Femininity is often used by this group of girls as a form of rebellion. Girls dress up, wear make-up and short skirts and often flaunt their femininity. Some have reputations for being sexually experienced and they pour scorn on the 'keenos', the girls who are careerists.

The third factor that alienates girls from school and learning is the behaviour of boys. Much of what turns even the formal educational process in a sexist direction is derived from the social dynamics of the classroom. As far as girls are concerned this is associated with the classroom behaviour of boys. Cheryll talks of boys:

> Well, I think of boys of that age, they're sort of putting you off and . . . You get people who are really influenced by the boys' presence. Some people just can't concentrate. You're always looking at the person behind you or around the corner who's flicking his pencil or talking to you or something.

The language of sexual abuse enables boys to define the school and its resources as part of their public sphere to the exclusion of girls. At one school, for example, there was a table-tennis craze, and the boys wanted to push the girls off the tables. The girls who refused to be pushed were called 'show-offs', not just by the boys but by other girls. They were regarded as sexually forward in standing up to the boys. Girls' participation in the classroom is equally unwelcome and they are at best ignored, or at worst ridiculed or put down.

> They don't take any notice of you when they're with their mates or they take the mickey out of you.

Much of a boys' group solidarity is based on collective denigration of girls who may even be their friends:

> They talk about our mates horribly, the ones they know are really good friends. They say they know for a fact that she is a slag and has been passed around the five of them. They say awful things when it's not true. Even when you walk along the street they scream at you.

Putting girls down is a daily part of classroom life:

> If he wants to borrow a ruler or something and we don't

give it to him 'cos we borrowed him something before, and he, like, calls you a prat. He says, 'All right, prat. You're so damned tight you won't give us anything.' So we go, 'That's right,' then every time he comes to the lesson they call you 'prat, prat' . . . 'Prat's sitting down on the chair,' 'Prat's got a ruler,' and all the rest of it. You don't have a chance.

Anti-school, Anti-work

The group most alienated from school is that of girls who reject both the learning process and any orientation to a career and at the same time do not focus their lives around school as a social environment. Most of these girls cannot wait to leave, get a job and in many cases are already heavily socialized into domestic labour and housework routines and see their future in marriage. Careena has no positive thoughts about school:

> When you're out of school, it's really good, it's so funny, nothing boring ever happens. It's just good . . . When you're in school it's horrible.

Jennifer and Cheryll agree:

> The one thing I really don't like about school is there's a lot of apathy. People are really apathetic. They just haven't got the energy to do anything. They just sit around, can't be bothered.

> I can't wait to leave. It's dragging on. It seems ages. I'm not really gonna take much more, y'know. I think you should be able to leave at fifteen if you want. I've got to wait another whole year. When I'm at school I'm sitting in lessons and I'll sit there talking about what I'd do if I was outside school. I make plans for the future.

The routine and repetitiveness of school were continually mentioned:

> School is very repetitive. You do the same thing every week. That's the thing I dislike most. On Monday you have history, Tuesday English, Wednesday something else. My sister who is in the second year wants to leave

already. So I said, 'Look, stick it out till the end of the third year, then start bunking off.'

It is these girls that are in the process of insulating themselves from career goals. Delamont (1980) argues that girls do not seem to realize that they will have to work for most of their lives in badly paid, unskilled jobs unless they leave school with qualifications, and seem 'blinded to the realities of the labour market by the rosy glow of romance'. Valerie knows she will have to work and is not romantic but considers low-paid work preferable to school:

> I mean, anything to do with school I hate. But if I was put in a supermarket or a café, I'd really enjoy it. 'Cos I'd be on the go, like, all the time. Like, when I used to work in a supermarket, I used to do stacking up, you didn't have to concentrate. It's like you were in a dream, really a daze. At school I sit there and I'm tired and a bit lazy and I get fed up. That's when I start answering the teachers back, which ain't much cop. Then your mum gets your bad report and thinks, 'Oh, after all I've done for you.' Then you say you're gonna be good this term and you're not. So you're in it, ain't you?

I have argued that it is not so much romance that puts girls off working for a career as the constraints of raising children and working whether married or not. Some girls are quite realistic about this. Sally, when asked what she sees herself doing in five years' time, replies:

> I don't see myself working actually. Either at home or queuing at the Labour Exchange, something like that ... By the time I'm a bit older, out of every hundred girls in every year at school, by the time they reach the third year, twenty out of a hundred are pregnant. A girl in my class she's got a baby who's a couple of months old. I don't see myself working.

The possibility of girls achieving very much in the public sphere was not taken seriously by most girls. Like the girls Mandy Llewellyn (1980) interviewed, some girls poured scorn

on the top-stream girls, who they considered had been hood-
winked, and they labelled them as 'keenos', 'stuck up', and
'snotty': 'Exams won't get them nowhere, they'll be out with
their prams next year – if anyone'll have 'em.' 'You see the
way they dress? – Wouldn't be seen dead like that.' 'Taint
never seen them with a lad' (Llewellyn 1980).

The relationship between this group of girls and teachers
is often antagonistic. Various forms of sexism among teachers is
a constant theme that alienated many girls from the school.
Sandy describes a teacher with sexist views as follows:

> This jewellery teacher. He believes the woman is just
> there for the home and nothing else. We often have
> arguments with him. We says women should have equal
> rights to men and he says, 'Not really – you don't have
> to say yes when we ask you to marry us.' It's because
> girls have been brought up to think they should do lots
> of work [in the house] and the boys are expecting us girls
> to do all the work, they expect their mums to do it and
> when they marry they expect the girls to do it.

This is not to say that girls sympathize with feminism. Some
girls find feminist teachers hard to accept. Marina criticizes a
teacher who argues that

> We have got to fight against men. It puts you off. Like *The
> Two Ronnies* 'Life of a Worm' – have you seen it? – It's like
> women do everything and men are absolute rubbish.

Outright sexism is described by a number of girls. A black
working-class girl speaks bitterly about the sexism she has
received from a teacher:

> He picks me out. 'Jenny,' he goes. I go, 'Yeah.' 'You little
> fucker.' 'What right have you to insult me?' He goes,
> 'What?' I was gonna kill him – if no teacher had come in that
> door, I swear it, I was really gonna beat him. I hate teachers
> like that. He's heard from another teacher that I'm cheeky
> so he goes, 'Oh Jenny, cheeky little cunt, ain't you?' . . . I
> can't stand people swearing at me.

Sometimes girls retaliate:

Our teacher called this girl a stupid bitch. All she's interested in is clothes. The girl got on her high horse and walloped the teacher. She got into bad trouble. The teacher denied it.

Of course not all teachers are like this:

Some teachers treat girls and boys the same. But it depends on what the teacher's like. Some of them think girls should do this and that, and some of them think they should be treated the same.

Teachers who are 'too chummy' and break the boundaries between the role of 'teacher' and 'pupil' are regarded with great suspicion by girls, quite rightly as teachers are not above abusing their authority over teenage girls. Sharon describes the type of teacher:

I hate teachers in this school, can't stand them, to me they're not teachers. When I first came to this school we had teachers who dressed up as if they was a teacher, y'know what I mean, like three-piece suit, tie, you know, they were strict. And the thing that made you learn in class was that you were afraid of them. If you didn't do your work you thought, he's gonna hit me or put me in detention. Through that you used to learn, you used to work. But now teachers are like the kids. I swear this is no joke. A teacher goes to me, 'You gotta fag?' I goes, 'No.' He goes, 'Why not? I would give you one.' I goes, 'I wouldn't ask you for one.' I wouldn't dare ask a teacher if he'd got a fag. In school, you know, a teacher goes to me, 'Have you gotta fag?' Two days ago . . . Before you know it all the teachers are going to go 'Gotta fag? Gotta fag?' Because they'd know if I'd given one teacher one. I think teachers shouldn't do that. They should try and stop us from smoking but they do it themselves.

Sharon is aware that the teacher is trying to develop familiarity here, and she is suspicious of his motives and wary of his advances.

Flirting and teasing can be used by teachers to maintain and perpetuate sex differences as Stanworth (1981) showed in her study of girls at a college of further education.

What determines which of these four courses are taken by girls through the education system? Obviously the type of school has an influence. Girls in single-sex schools, where the presence of boys as a disturbing factor does not apply, are more career oriented. We have seen that class is also important. Middle-class girls are more likely to be career oriented and working-class girls more likely to be already involved in domestic chores at the expense of school and homework. Working-class girls are likely to receive less support from home and to face all sorts of educational disadvantages. The girls are very conscious of class as manifested by accent, lifestyle and money. One reason why working-class girls lead more restricted lives is of course financial.

> My friends they have to face the fact that one week they have no pocket-money so they aren't able to do something whereas the others can always sponge money if they want it. They never have to say, 'Well I've got no money, I can't go somewhere,' whereas we say, 'Oh, I'm skint this week,' or, 'It's my week for being poor this week.' Then the next week you'll buy her a coffee or something – they [the middle-class girls] don't seem to be like that. I think some girls are very over-protected.

Belinda thinks class is very important but often disguises ambiguities:

> I think class is too important. Everyone's sort of classed as 'Oh, we're the snobs,' then there's Tania's group, they're all from the East End. They think of us as the brainy ones and Tania's group are all going to do CSEs, but I'm doing CSEs.

Along with class there is the overpowering pressure of gender stereotypes, which act on all girls. The weight of all the pressures we have looked at throughout this study affects the girls' performance at school. The ever-present power of the 'slag' category is not restricted to girls' social life as opposed to their educational performance. But the two aspects, it is worth emphasizing again, do not just exist side by side, they are in interaction: the social dynamics of the classroom and the playground influence the aspirations and performance of pupils in the formal learning situation. The aspects of the control of girls through 'slag' that we have looked at in other chapters thus have a crucial bearing on actual educational performance. What happens to girls is therefore determined within certain boundaries by the very fact of their being girls and not by their being pupils or working-class or academically successful. The slag/drag dichotomy or the too tight/too loose distinction is one that is used by groups of girls against each other. As Sandy says,

> In class, in school – people are always calling you a slut – you're a tramp or a snob ... It's probably 'cos we think that they look down on us and they probably think we look down on them, you just assume this is what happens and the minute you see them, a wall builds up and you don't want to break it down. You just accept it.

To what extent are schools addressing the problem of the denigration of girls and pervasiveness of verbal sexual abuse? In the eighties we saw the emergence of equal opportunities policies in schools and colleges across the country. The aim of these policies was initially to encourage women to move into privileged and senior positions in existing educational institutions where they are so under-represented, but with the decline of single-sex schooling and move to comprehensive education the number of female heads has actually declined (*Times Educational Supplement* 1983). More recently equal opportunity initiatives have focused on adapting the curriculum and drawing up policies in regard to sexual harassment and sex education.

How Far Have Girls' Attitudes Changed?

All the schools where the research was undertaken were attempting to combat gender discrimination – one with a girls-only maths group – and all had integrated discussions of sexism into the sex-education curriculum. In this section I shall look at some of the girls' views about women's liberation and the way girls cope with sexism from boys.

Middle-class girls were more likely to be critical of chauvinism and the double standard. As one sexually experienced mature girl about to start an A-level course in science explains:

> Some girls have different attitudes. The girls who are thinking of getting engaged already are the girls who talk about sluts and talk about people who sleep around and really look down on them. And the boys that they know wouldn't touch them with a bargepole but it doesn't really involve my sort of circle. I suppose that's more about being liberated. The boys who go down the pub are the sort who sneer at girls who sleep around. But the sort who talk to girls as friends and take them down to the pub and sort of have a good night out with the girls and the boys together not really thinking about what sex they are, they're the sort ... They take it more lightly and if they can sleep around why shouldn't the girls. They're more likely to think of it like that. Which is really only fair. 'Cos you don't get girls who say, 'Oh that boy's a real whore, don't go near him, he's dirt.'

Other girls agree that the double standard of sexual morality is weakening:

> There's all this nastiness about – a man who sleeps around is just a man who sleeps around and a woman who sleeps around is a real slag and you've got to keep away from her. But I think in my circles that sort of thing is fading away. Obviously, things like that are fading away more and more over the years. People are out for more sexual equality. Although boys will probably want more sex than girls, but I don't see any reason why [girls] shouldn't have sex. It's not all that much of a big step.

Girls who express such progressive views are unusual, however, and for most girls, even those who are aware of the double standard (and by no means all girls are), to resist the categorization is difficult, as the label attacks girls individually and it is as individuals that they are left to resist.

Some boys, from both middle- and working-class groups,

express comparable views. Toby, for example, a middle-class fifteen-year-old who lives alone with his mother, argues:

> TOBY I would never call a girl a slag. It's unfair. If a boy goes out with lots of girls then he'll think he's OK, but if a girl goes out with lots of boys it's not OK. It's a bit old-fashioned.
>
> Q *Why isn't it OK for a girl to go out with lots of boys?*
>
> People don't think it's OK, they think she should stay at home.

Mike also does not agree with acting 'macho':

> Not all boys try to act macho and tough. I mean, I try not to go around looking like a macho man, girls think it's daft. If you go around trying to look really tough another tough boy might come up to you and start trying to look tougher and start a fight. Personally I think it looks daft.

When it comes to discussing women's liberation his views are refreshingly enlightened:

> Depending on what they're after as such, it could be a very good thing. If they're after equality, then that's good, but if they're after doing what they say men are doing now, taking power, then I think that's bad as they are going against their own views. So you see the point is that one sex shouldn't have all the power. If they're going after power for themselves, then that's going against their principles.

When asked what evidence he has for women going for power, the reply is:

> Power-crazy people – I don't want to mention names, but there was a Prime Minister once upon a time.

Studies of Teacher Attitudes

There have been few studies of teacher attitudes to sexism or of how teachers are socialized into the occupation. Most teachers are from lower-middle-class and upper-working-class backgrounds, where sex roles tend to be most traditional and segregated (see Delamont 1990). Most recruits to teaching have had and will have conventional ideas about sex roles and little is done to change this during training (Equal Opportunities Commission 1989). Even student teachers who were aware of sexism on their training courses failed to see it when in schools (Skelton and Hanson 1989). One of the few studies on teacher-training courses found that the course content was laden with assumptions about male and female pupils, all of which became self-fulfilling prophecies (Good 1973). It is important to look at teachers' attitudes to understand why they fail to intervene. There is evidence that teachers react with hostility or reluctance to anti-sexist intervention strategies and that the implementation of equal opportunities seems to be left to isolated individual teachers (Riddell 1989).

Unfortunately, as we have seen, with the decline of single-sex schooling and the move to mixed comprehensive education, the total number of female heads in schools in Britain has actually declined. There is mounting evidence that mixed schooling has increased the sexism that girls are subjected to (see Mahony 1985, Weiner 1985, Askew and Ross 1988). Sexism may be on the agenda, but many men and some women are hostile or indifferent to bringing about changes to reduce sex discrimination. There is also evidence from a number of studies that young girls are sexually harassed and sometimes frightened out of their wits by gangs of boys. Much of this violence is taken for granted by girls and teachers alike. Just as it never occurs to girls in my study to say, 'How dare they call us slags,' Halson describes how it never seemed to occur to the young women to say, 'How dare they assault us.' All they say is, 'It's horrible,' 'It's embarrassing,' 'I don't care. I've got over it now,' 'You can't do nothin' about it,' (Halson 1989).

Effects of Education Initiatives

In Britain the last five years have seen the enactment of a number of government initiatives in the field of education, some of which have been directed at gender inequalities. These initiatives have been concerned with encouraging girls to enter non-traditional areas. It could be argued that the aim is to fit girls into boys' education. National research projects such as the Girls into Science and Technology (GIST 1981–4) and the School Council Sex Differentiation Project (1981–3) documented inequalities, and the Genderwatch project in Merton was set up to produce materials to counteract discrimination.

The first major gender initiative in education was created by the Manpower Services Commission (MSC) set up in 1973 to be responsible for the promotion of training for employment. In 1984 the MSC identified sex-stereotyping as an obstacle to educational progress and announced that with respect to the Technical and Vocational Educational Initiative (TVEI) a criterion for funding would be the availability of initiatives to pupils regardless of sex or race and care should be taken to avoid sex-stereotyping (MSC 1984). Cynthia Cockburn who assessed the progress made by the MSC in enabling young women to cross gender contrary areas of training and work confirmed the pattern of sex-stereotyping in youth-training programmes and identified two key factors that needed to be recognized:

• The significance of 'gender culture' – a large feminization was required in order to create an environment in which young women could make 'really free choices'.

• The significance of the specification of occupations that enables males to create and preserve their own space and then elevate its status.

She recommended as strategies single-sex streaming in some or all the sessions, supportive training policies, women teachers in technical subjects and intensive work with young men on sexism (Cockburn 1987).

Ann Marie Wolpe (1988), whose research is based on years of participant observation in classrooms and in the school generally, along with verbatim quotations from interviews with pupils, teachers and parents, concludes that to effect changes in girls' education requires drastic changes in the education system, among other things; the system needs systematically to be reviewed and restructured.

The Way Forward

Much of the confused thinking about sexuality and the failure to acknowledge the way conceptions of masculinity and femininity are socially rather than biologically constructed stem from essentialist ideas about some behaviour being 'natural' and therefore unalterable. It is regarded as natural for girls to be attracted to boys, unnatural for girls to have intense relationships with the same sex; natural for them to undertake if not enjoy domesticity, natural for boys to be allowed out and girls to be kept in, natural for a girl to be 'chatted up' and made to feel uncomfortable and to want to get married and have children, but unnatural to want a career that would conflict with marriage or to put her main energies into sport or creative activities. Above all a girl is expected to put others before herself and to be caring and unselfish. In the same vein it is considered natural for men to put themselves first, natural for them to be promiscuous, natural for the woman to try and 'catch' a man and entice him into marriage, unnatural for a woman to live without a man, natural for a man to hit his wife if she is disobedient or allegedly unfaithful. Men are not seen to have a responsibility for caring either for children or the elderly. On the contrary, it is regarded as unmanly to be involved in such activities.

The idea that masculine and feminine behaviour is 'natural' is very difficult to challenge as it is embedded in common sense. I remember when my daughter was young, her grandfather saw her playing with a broom. He commented, 'There you are, you can see how feminine and domesticated she is going to be when she grows up – a proper little woman.' When my son picked up the broom he suggested to him that he was 'riding to battle on a white stallion'. The difficulty of challenging such assumptions is that evidence for naturalness is usually drawn from the observation that some behaviour is more typical of girls than boys. Even when this is the case (and often, as in this incident, it is due more to selective perception than to what actually occurs), and girls are found to be doing more housework and participating less in sport, this merely shows how effectively social norms work. What is suggested by the attribution of naturalness is that the behaviour is unchangeable and should be left untouched.

Sexual behaviour is formed by powerful social discourses rather than biology. This refutes the idea of unequal relations between the sexes as natural, yet both girls and boys usually take it for granted that the differences between the sexes are biological, as 'common sense' dictates. The position I take in this book is that essentialist ideas are themselves social constructions that need to be challenged. It is no more natural for a girl to do housework than for a boy, or for a boy to learn to care for children or to take responsibility for his sexual behaviour which, contrary to 'common sense' notions, is not more 'uncontrollable' than a girl's. For girls to enter the public sphere on equal terms to boys, they need to be seen not as sex objects but as human beings. The evidence for this rests on the growing number of women who are contesting their inferiority.

Not only parents but teachers can be seen to collude in 'essentialism': they often do not contest outright sexist abuse from little boys on the grounds that it is natural. Valerie Walkerdine in her critique of the application of psychoanalytic educational pedagogy to nursery school describes how a woman teacher is 'brought down to size' by a tiny boy calling her a 'cunt'. The teacher, who has been taught that free expression is all-important in teaching young children, only belatedly and then very gently rebukes the child. When asked why she responded in this way to such demeaning sexual abuse she replied: 'Those kind of expressions are quite normal for this age ... As long as they're not being too silly or bothering anybody, it's just natural and should be left ... Coming out with that kind of expression is very natural'

(Walkerdine 1990:6). She fails to see how this produces and facilitates her own collusion in her oppression. The teacher is rendered powerless to resist the power of the boys.

Common sense means that it is difficult to question all sorts of ideas. This is clear in the way that housework is considered to be natural for girls. How are girls to be taught to challenge ideas that are so taken for granted?

Jane Gaskell's study of Canadian girls at school came to very similar conclusions to this research. She found that the girls' view of men, masculinity and the limits of acceptable or natural male behaviour has changed little:

[Girls'] construction of masculinity is rooted in an ideology which suggests that what men are like is what men must be like. Biological explanations of the difference between men and women and the domestic ideology's construction of the special nature of men and women shape their perceptions . . . Their perceptions are validated by their experiences of patriarchal family structures. They have not seen men in domestic roles. Their fathers, brothers and boyfriends do housework only as a special favour, for a woman (Gaskell 1992:79).

Studies of white girls in Britain (Mirza 1992) and in Canada (Gaskell 1992) portray girls as not expecting to be the main earner, taking it for granted that child-rearing and a lower earning capacity will combine to force them to give up work while their children are young, even though this is not necessarily what they wanted. In an Australian study of Melbourne girls (Wyn 1990), girls express similar views. They are not romantic about marriage and relationships with men but see marriage and particularly child-rearing as an important feature of their future life. Bringing up children is an immeasurably fulfilling goal. The difficulty lies in boys being brought up not to carry equal responsibility, to enable girls to combine work and childcare, but to be the sole breadwinner, in charge of the household. They are being brought up, both at home and at school, for a world that no longer exists. Even more damaging is the relegation of these tasks to feminine and therefore inferior work. The result is women who are struggling to take on two roles, and men who have outmoded views of the relations between the sexes. Education does not appear to be concerned with this vital issue.

Conclusions

Virginia Woolf was sceptical of the idea that education could liberate women. On the outbreak of the Second World War, in *Three Guineas* (1938), she sees education not as the road to freedom but as a training in domination, in élitism and in militarism. She argues that the values that led Germany into war are mirrored in our own educational system. She then poses the crucial question of whether women would want to join men in what she calls 'the procession of men'. Do women want to wear wigs and gowns, she asks, to make money, administer justice, dress in military uniform, with gold lace on their breasts, swords at their sides? The question she then puts is just as relevant today:

We are here to ask ourselves certain questions and they are very important questions, and we have very little time in which to answer them. The questions that we have to ask and to answer about that procession during this moment of transition are so important that they may well change the lives of all men and women for ever. For we have to ask ourselves, here and now, do we wish to join that procession, or don't we? On what terms shall we join the procession? Above all, where is it leading us, the procession of educated men? (Woolf 1938)

Woolf argues that education is based on male experience and roles to the exclusion of feminine experience, encompassing the qualities and responsibilities of caring and of sensibility.

There does seem to be evidence that at least some boys are being made aware by girls of the inequality and sexism around them, and to be opposing such views. Many boys are now helping, if only minimally, with the housework, and a significant number of girls are beginning to challenge their relegation to housework and the home. In the next chapter I propose that the statutory provision for sex education and the introduction of the common curriculum could provide a forum for challenging essentialist ideas and introducing a critique of patriarchal culture in the way proposed by Virginia Woolf.

The whole ethos of education with its emphasis on competitiveness and instrumentalism needs to be challenged. The hierarchical structure of our educational institutions, not merely in terms of the institutional structure but also in terms of the hierarchy of human attributes, needs questioning. We need to educate girls and boys for a society where gender divisions are less relevant and women and men share in paid work and caring.

Overall the girls in this research do not subscribe to the idea that woman's place is only in the home. They are indignant that their brothers are required to undertake less housework than they do. Much has been said about quiet, submissive girls in studies of education. This does not fit in with Jerry, a sixteen-year-old boy I interviewed. Girls are rowdy, he assured me, and the idea that they are quiet is:

> Illusions. We have some of the noisiest girls in our class. We generally don't get to leave school until late because the girls won't keep quiet. They are very, very noisy.

Notes

1. The phrase appears in the Hansard report documenting discrimination against women in all areas of life, politics, the economy, the law, universities and business. At the launch of the report at the House of Commons, when asked by a Member of Parliament what was to happen to the men who would be displaced if the representation of women in positions of authority were improved, Lady Howe, who chaired the Committee, answered 'Don't misunderstand me, I am not in favour of positive action.'

2. As I write this book my eighty-six-year-old father has sent me a load of darning to do, in indignation that I am not spending more time with him.

Bibliography

Acker, S. (ed.), 1989, *Teachers, Gender and Careers*, Falmer Press
Arnot, M., 1984, 'How shall we educate our sons?', in Deem, R. (ed.), *Education Reconsidered*, Open University Press

Askew, S., and Ross, C., 1988, *Boys Don't Cry: Boys and Sexism in Education*, Oxford University Press

Beddoe, D., 1983, *Discovering Women's History*, Pandora Press

Brah, A., and Minhas, R., 1985, 'Structural Racism or Cultural Difference: Schooling for Asian Girls', in Weiner, G. (ed.), *Just a Bunch of Girls*, Oxford University Press

Cockburn, C., 1987, *Two Track Training*, Macmillan

Cockburn, C., 1991, *In the Way of Women*, Macmillan

Coleman, J., and Hendry, L., 1990 *The Nature of Adolescence*, 2nd edition, Routledge and Kegan Paul

Deem, R., 1984, *Coeducation Reconsidered*, Open University Press

Delamont, S., 1980, *Sex Roles and the School*, Methuen

Delamont, S., 1990, *Sex Roles and the School*, 2nd edition, Routledge and Kegan Paul

Equal Opportunities Commission, 1989, Formal Investigation Report: Initial Teacher Training in England and Wales, Manchester, EOC 73

Evans, G., 1980, 'Those Loud Black Girls', in Spender, D., and Sarah, E. (eds.), *Learning to Lose*, 2nd edition, Women's Press

Fogelman, K., 1976, *Britain's Sixteen-Year-Olds*, National Children's Bureau

Fordham, S., and Ogbu, J., 1986, 'Black Students' School Success: Coping with the Burden of Acting White', in *The Urban Review*, 18 (3), pp. 176–206

Fuller, H., 1980, 'Black Girls in a London Comprehensive School', in Deem, R. (ed.), *Schooling for Women's Work*, Routledge and Kegan Paul

Gaskell, J., 1992, *Gender Matters: From School to Work*, Oxford University Press

Good, T.L., 1973, 'Teacher Expectations', in Berliner, D., and Rosenshine, B. (eds.), *Talks to Teachers*, Teachers College Press 26

Griffin, C., 1985, *Typical Girls*, Routledge and Kegan Paul

Halson, J., 1989, 'The Sexual Harassment of Young Women', in Holly, L. (ed.), *Girls and Sexuality: Teaching and Learning*, Oxford University Press

Hansard Society Commission, 1990, Report on Women at the Top

Llewellyn, M., 1980, 'Studying Girls at School: The Implications of Confusion', in Deem, R. (ed.), *Schooling for Women's Work*, Routledge and Kegan Paul

Mahony, P., 1985, *Schools for the Boys? Coeducation Reassessed*, Hutchinson

Marshall, J., 1983, 'Developing Anti-Sexist Education', *International Journal of Political Education*, 16, No. 2

McRobbie, A., 1978, 'Working-Class Girls and the Culture of Femininity', in *Women Take Issue*, Hutchinson

Mirza, H., 1992, *Young, Female and Black*, Routledge

Payne, I., 1980, 'Sexist Ideology and Education', in Spender, D., and Sarah, E. (eds.), *Learning to Lose*, Women's Press

Phoenix, A., 1987, 'Theories of Gender and Black Families', in Weiner, G., and Arnot, M. (eds.), *Gender under Scrutiny*, Hutchinson

Reay, D., 1990, 'Working with Boys', in *Gender and Education*, Vol. 2, No. 3

Riddell, S., 1989, 'It's Nothing to do with Me: Teachers' Views and Gender Divisions in the Curriculum', in Acker, S. (ed.), *Teachers, Gender and Careers*, Falmer Press

Skelton, C., and Hanson, J., 1989, 'Schooling the Teachers', in Acker, S. (ed.), *Teachers, Gender and Careers*, Falmer Press

Spender, D., 1982, *Invisible Women*, Writers and Readers Press

Stanworth, M., 1981, *Gender and Schooling: A Study of Sexual Divisions in the Classroom*, Hutchinson

Stone, M., 1985, *The Education of the Black Child*, Fontana

Times Educational Supplement, 1983, 'Protest over Head's Appointment', June 24 1983, p. 1

Walkerdine, V., 1990, *Schoolgirl Fictions*, Verso

Ward, J., 1990, 'Racial Identity: Formation and Transformation', in Gilligan, C., et al. (eds.), *Making Connections*, Harvard University Press

Weiner, G., 1985, *Just a Bunch of Girls*, Oxford University Press

Willis, P., 1977, *Learning to Labour*, Saxon House

Wilson, A., 1978, *Finding a Voice*, Virago

Wollstonecraft, Mary, 1792, *On the Vindication of the Rights of Women*, reissued 1988, W. W. Norton

Wolpe, A. M., 1988, *Within School Walls: The Role of Discipline, Sexuality and the Curriculum*, Routledge and Kegan Paul

Woolfe, V., 1938, *Three Guineas*, Hogarth Press

Wyn, J., 1990, 'Working-Class Girls and Educational Outcomes: Is Self-Esteem an Issue', in Kenway, J., and Willis, S. (eds.), *Hearts and Minds: Self-Esteem and the Schooling of Girls*, Falmer Press

Chapter 5
Sex Education

BRIAN A girl and a boy go out to get a baby. A boy and a boy go out to get AIDS.
JIMMY AIDS is punishment for someone who goes fucking around.
MIKE You can get AIDS from anyone.
JIMMY You can't catch it from women.
MIKE Yes you can. People think AIDS is only for queers. You can get it from a blood transfusion, from women, from sperm.

(Group discussion, sixteen-year-old boys)

The question of sex education is one of the most highly sensitive and controversial educational issues precisely because it deals with the area that is excluded from the education system, the area that is geared not to prepare boys and girls for work but for their wider responsibilities. The educational system is a set of institutions concerned with what has been called secondary socialization. It is the family where primary socialization is presumed to take place, where people are seen as whole human beings and accepted with all their weaknesses and foibles, concerned with community rather than with bureaucracy and instrumentalism. Therefore there is a fundamental tension and ambiguity about introducing questions of the body and sexuality, issues of responsibility and moral choice, quite apart from unmentionable topics such as menstruation and childbirth, into the classroom.[1]

In Britain the national curriculum now requires pupils aged eleven to fourteen to understand the processes of conception in human beings, know about the physical and emotional changes that take place during adolescence and understand the need to have a responsible attitude to sexual behaviour. They must also now study the ways in which the healthy functioning of the human body may be affected by HIV (The Health of the Nation 1992). With the introduction of the national curriculum there is little space allocated to non-foundation subjects, so sex education is still patchy in many schools.

I consider the problems that arise from this and the effects of the AIDS crisis and the introduction of a national framework for the provision of sex education as part of the national curriculum introduced in 1988. I then outline three different political views of sex education: the conservative, the liberal and the feminist. A feminist approach involves questioning the social inequality between girls and boys and introducing sex education within the context of the sexism so rampant within social relations in school. Finally I will consider the obstacles to implementing sex-education policies and the extent to which schools are succeeding in preparing both girls and boys for their roles as sexual partners and parents in a world that is undergoing rapid change. The issue of sex education will not go away precisely because we are living at a time when rapid changes are irreversibly re-shaping the relationships between the sexes and between home and work. To put the discussion into context, I will begin by considering the impact of changes in sexual practices over the last decades.

Changes in Sexual Practice

To what extent have girls been liberated by the changes in sexual practices among adolescents over the past fifty years? The period following the Second World War has seen a continuing lowering of the age of the onset of menstruation together with significant changes in premarital sexual behaviour. In the USA (see Voydanoff and Donnelly 1990), Europe and Britain (Farrell 1978) there has been a trend towards earlier and more frequent sexual intercourse among adolescents of both sexes. Farrell's work, which followed the so-called era of sexual liberation of the late sixties and early seventies, suggests that for adolescent girls at least these changes are less far-reaching than imagined. The rise in teen-age pregnancy and transmission of sexually transmitted dis-eases (STD) are much lower than the media-inspired moral panics might lead us to suppose, promiscuity is rare and teenagers are no more likely to have a casual sexual relation-ship than thirty years ago. As Judith Bury comments: 'Young people may become sexually active at a younger age, but their sexual behaviour is still regulated by such traditional values as love, fidelity, partnership, marriage and the family' (Bury 1984).

None the less, some significant changes have taken place. The availability of the birth-control pill since the 1960s has made childbirth a real choice; the prejudice against unmarried mothers keeping their children is immeasurably less than twenty years ago and unmarried girls are increasingly opting to keep their children. The possibility of existing on state benefits must have contributed to this. In the 1990s, therefore, in the UK, pre-marital sex is common (Ford 1989; Ford and Morgan 1989:171). This is not only facilitated by the greater availability of abortion (following the Abortion Act of 1967) and of contraception, but also by advances in penicillin and antibiotic treatments for venereal disease. The idea of 'a woman's right to choose' is applied by feminists not only to whether or not to give birth but to other realms of behaviour. The proportion of illegitimate births increased from 5 per cent in 1950 to 25.6 per cent in 1988 (Social Trends 1990). The meaning of illegitimacy has changed, following its dramatic rise since the 1960s, culminating in its abolition in the Legiti-macy Act 1988. There is now far more tolerance of different types of sexual behaviour.

The changes of the 1980s and 1990s may not have made sexual relations easier to cope with for girls. There is less pressure to get married but more pressure to have sex. The marriage rate among teenagers has decreased both in Britain and the USA. In the USA the decline has been dramatic among white teenagers, and black teenagers rarely marry. In

1983 four out of ten births to white teenagers were out of wedlock against nine out of ten to blacks (Vinovskis 1988:29). Birth-control and abortions are more available and the stigma of becoming pregnant has decreased.

In the USA the rate of adolescent pregnancy and child-bearing is higher than in other industrialized countries. In 1981 the pregnancy rate was twice that of England and Wales, France and Canada, three times that of Sweden and six times that of the Netherlands (Voydanoff and Donnelly 1990). More than half the pregnancies are unintended. One in two of these is terminated by abortion. Most women obtaining abortions are young: 58 per cent are under twenty-five; 26 per cent are teenagers. This is one reason why it is likely that President Bush's anti-abortion stand may well have lost him votes in the 1992 presidential election. Since more than half the marriages in the USA break up, and the average length of marriage is ten years, many women are bringing up children on their own. Abortion is therefore a crucial issue for women. *A Woman's Book of Choices* (Chalker and Downer 1992), which tells women how they can terminate one another's pregnancies by menstrual extraction, may prove to be a landmark in the attempt of women to gain control over reproduction.

In Britain, the assumed problem of teenage pregnancy still attracts widespread media attention and exaggerated publicity. Teenage fertility has in fact been declining throughout the developed world. Sue Sharpe (1987) points out births to teenagers in Britain fell in the 1970s and early 1980s. This fall has been explained by the greater use of contraceptives by teenagers, particularly those over sixteen and the rise in the number of abortions. In 1984 the sixteen to nineteen age group had a higher abortion rate than any other. Pregnancies among the youngest teenagers are the most likely to end in abortion; one in four nineteen-year-olds, but three in four of those aged fifteen or less ended their pregnancies (Francome 1986). In the late 1980s teenage pregnancy rates rose slightly owing to a small rise in the number of girls having babies. Overall however the number of teenage mothers is still small and British research suggests that most of them manage very well with the help of their mothers (Phoenix 1990, Sharpe 1987:3).

A major change in the last five years is that AIDS is now seen as a threat not only to homosexuals and drug abusers, but also to at least some sectors of the heterosexual population. Since reporting began in 1982 a total of 5,684 AIDS cases (5,295 males, 353 females) have been reported in the UK, of whom 3,527 (62 per cent) are known to have died (British Youth Council 1992). The majority of new adult cases continues to consist of homosexual men, but recent figures confirm a steady spread of the disease among heterosexuals, which has now reached 25 per cent of the total number of cases (Public Health Laboratory Service March 1992), though this is not as great as was predicted some years ago.

Research on women and AIDS is still inadequate; two recent contributions concentrate on providing basic relevant information for women about AIDS and advice on safe-sex practices (Patton and Kelly 1987; Richardson 1987). The 15–34 age band accounts for 61 per cent of full-blown female AIDS cases, but only 42 per cent of males; the figures for reported HIV infection are 83 per cent for women in this age band and 62 per cent for men (British Youth Council 1992). It is not clear why this is so, though it could be a result of young women being more at risk of infection due to the greater permeability of the vagina. The higher age of male sufferers would be accounted for by the higher risk for homosexuals. A question of great concern in regard to the spread of the disease among young women is the risk HIV-positive mothers have of passing the virus on to their offspring during pregnancy. The child can be infected in the womb, during birth as a result of contact with infected blood or vaginal secretions and possibly after birth through breast milk. Studies show that between 30 per cent and 50 per cent of all

HIV-positive mothers pass the virus on to their children (Hauer 1989).

One effect of the impact of AIDS has been to promote far greater discussion of sex than has ever occurred before: until a few years ago 'condom' was a forbidden word on the BBC in Britain, and 'safe sex' was unheard of. Feminist critiques have focused on the prevalent male-oriented definition of hetero-sexuality and heterosexual practice. Penetrative sex, the hallmark of the male definition of heterosexual practice, has been identified as a major contributor to the spread of AIDS. Practices described as safe sex refer to non-penetrative sex; kissing, cuddling, cunnilingus and mutual masturbation are being advocated in public-health campaigns and so are enter-ing the public discourse on sexuality, though there is little evidence that young heterosexuals are adopting such practices or that sex is any less focused on penetration.

Few studies of sexual behaviour existed in Britain until the threat of HIV infection led to studies into heterosexual life-styles, but over the past five years a number of studies have provided a great deal more information about sexual practices than has ever been available before. In a study undertaken in Bristol during 1988, of 400 young people between the ages of sixteen and twenty-one three broad types of philosophies were identified. First, traditional–restrictive, in which intercourse is reserved for marriage; second, liberal–romantic, in which intercourse is reserved for a steady relationship, and third, casual–recreational, in which intercourse outside a steady rela-tionship is acceptable (Ford 1991).

In this study nearly half of sixteen-year-olds had engaged in sexual intercourse, rising to 90 per cent of twenty-one-year-olds. Fifty-one per cent of the sixteen- to nineteen-year-olds he studied had had two or more partners. One-fifth of the sample condoned intercourse outside a steady relationship. In a much larger study in the USA, Zelnick and Kantner (1980) found a very similar picture. By 1979, 48.5 per cent of seventeen-year-old girls were sexually experienced. Among nineteen-year-olds

69 per cent had had sexual intercourse. This study found a marked difference between white and black girls; 73.3 per cent of the latter had had a sexual experience by the age of seventeen. Class has also been found to be relevant, in so far as working-class boys in Britain have been found to be more sexually experienced than boys of other classes (Farrell 1978). In the USA the greatest changes in attitudes and behaviour have occurred among liberal white middle-class boys and girls (Conger and Petersen 1984).

A number of surveys have indicated that not only is pre-marital sex now common, but that casual sex is increasing. The study carried out by Nick Ford at Exeter University (Ford 1991) found that 25 per cent of girls and 52 per cent of boys thought sex was all right outside a steady relationship. Only 3 per cent of girls and boys thought it should be saved for marriage. He also found that the majority of girls preferred hugging and kissing to intercourse. Fifty-eight per cent of sixteen-year-olds said they had had intercourse.

One shortcoming of most studies of sexual behaviour among young people is the failure to examine what sexual behaviour means to young people. Christine Farrell (1978), in her otherwise excellent study of how adolescents come to learn about sex, regards as entirely unproblematic what the experience of sex actually is. The whole question of how sexual relations control and constrain social life is missed.

Girls face an irreconcilable contradiction in regard to sex. They are under pressure to be seen as competent and confident sexually but not as 'slags', and it is a fine line to tread. Sex is a difficult area for everyone; for young women it's even harder. The boys in my research do not on the whole envisage marrying virgins. When asked in a group discussion whether they would mind having a girlfriend who was sexually experienced, they reply:

>BOY 1 Well, it's OK she's been touched by someone else.
>BOY 3 What, not like a packet of frozen peas?

BOY 2 So you can touch them before anyone else?

BOY 3 So you can put a mark on the chart on the wall?

BOY 2 Like truck drivers?

Q *Would you like your future wife to have sexual experience?*

BOY 3 You can't find a woman who hasn't had sexual experience. Not round here you can't, not in London.

I asked girls what they get out of their sexual relationships. Few of the girls spoke about sexual experience as pleasurable. They are aware that they have a great deal more freedom than their mothers, but they experience sex as an anti-climax and, as we shall see in the chapter on violence, often feel pressured into it. Take Miranda's account of her friend Sarah's experience of losing her virginity on a one-night stand:

It happens a lot. I've got a friend called Sarah who went to the Lyceum for the Greatest Disco in Town and I know she was a virgin. She went there and a kid decided that he really wanted to sleep with her and he said: 'Well I'm not going to go out with you if you don't.' So she did. I could never do that. Never ever. I'd just turn round and say, 'Forget it if you're like that.' Just walk off. But she didn't. She lost him the following day anyway.

When asked how she felt afterwards, Miranda replies:

I think she feels it was a waste. She didn't enjoy it and she was pressured into it and now it's gone. If I was in her situation and that happened to me I think I'd just be so down.

More optimistically there is some evidence that young women are gaining confidence. This is reflected in girls' magazines, which have radically changed in the last two decades with the decline of photo love stories around which many of the girls' magazines were marketed, where female passivity and traditional sex-role stereotyping took on a heightened form. In her analysis of *Jackie* and *Just Seventeen* McRobbie (1991) indicates how these love narratives disappeared in the

1980s as a result of readers informing the editors that they thought they were insulting and silly. Stories have since become far more realistic.

Lesbian girls have been ignored in most of the surveys of young people. A Canadian report (Lesbian and Gay Youth 1988) found that young lesbians and homosexuals are faced by pressure and hostility which leads to problem behaviour such as drug and alcohol abuse, delinquency, heterosexual promiscuity and pregnancy (as a last attempt to prove their heterosexuality). One-third of the young people interviewed reported dating members of the opposite sex in order to conceal their sexual orientation. Not only pupils but lesbian teachers face harassment both on account of their lesbianism and their gender which makes it very difficult for them to provide role models for girls (see Squirrell 1989). They stress the importance of preparing teachers to confront the name-calling and harassment in schools.

Similar distress was reported in a small survey carried out by the London Gay Teenage Group (Trenchard and Warren 1984). The horrified responses of parents who are told by their sons and daughters that they are gay or lesbian are graphically depicted. As one sixteen-year-old said:

[My mother's] first reaction was 'You'd better go to the doctor about it.' This was followed by, 'How disgusting, keep away from me' – as if homosexuality was contagious. Now she thinks that just because I like girls, I must either hate men or want to be a man (neither of which is true). I think she's hoping that I'll grow out of it, but I can't see this happening (I don't want to, either) (Trenchard and Warren 1984).

Boys in my research differed in their views of gays:
  BOY 3 I don't feel hatred against gays, I just feel a bit uneasy.
  Q *What would happen if a boy admitted to being gay?*
  BOY 2 If he was West Indian he'd probably get beaten by his West Indian friends and kicked out of his clan. In

a group of normal London kids they'd take the mickey out of him and want nothing to do with him no more, an outcast. Then the rest, another group, say it was all right but deep down inside they'd want nothing to do with him.

BOY 3 There are people who genuinely aren't prejudiced.

The introduction of information on AIDS in sex education provides an opportunity for teachers to raise the whole issue of homophobia. In my research lesbians were frequently associated with women's lib and many girls expressed marked prejudice:

Have you seen them? Two girls walking along, one of them's got cufflinks on and everything, just like a man. I think that's terrible – I think it's disgusting.

Poofs I can tolerate, but lesbians I can't. I suppose because it's my own sex.

Fear of seduction by lesbian girls is a constant theme – astonishing in the light of the real harassment that girls experience from boys in their day-to-day life:

Maybe we feel threatened by them – so we think to ourselves, 'Oh, my god, maybe if they tried to drag me into that thing.'

I think they'd start kind of threatening you, hassling you.

If a close friend came out as a lesbian, one girl says,

I wouldn't talk to her as much as I used to, not because I didn't like her as much, but because I'd be threatened by her.

In the 1960s and 1970s, while the liberalization of sexuality and more open discussion about sex could be seen as important gains, some women were aware of certain disadvantages that came with this new licence. The availability of the pill, for example, made it more difficult for women to refuse sex. Adrienne Rich (1980) in *Against Compulsory Heterosexuality* outlined the hazards of sexual expression under a patriarchy where girls and women are not on an equal footing to men and sexual expression takes place on male terms. Rich argues that the whole notion of 'consent' is questionable in a society that enforces heterosexuality and female submission on girls. In Britain the contradictions in acting out oppressive patriarchal relations of domination and subordination in relationships has been widely debated. Research on female pleasure in the USA (for example the Hite Reports 1976, 1988) concluded that many women still achieve limited gratification which can be attributed to such factors as the difficulties they experience in negotiating the nature of their sexual interactions with male partners and the identification of sex with penetration. A high proportion of women had never experienced orgasm. This latter research relates for the most part to older women and little is known about the attitudes and practices of girls who have recently become sexually active. *The Hite Report on Women and Love*, the culmination of the Hite report trilogy on sexuality, concluded: 'The biggest problem is not women's lack of financial independence or men's absence from domestic work, but men's reluctance to talk about personal thoughts and feelings' (Hite 1988).

After conducting a survey of 4,500 women, Shere Hite reported that most women were distressed and despairing about the continued refusal of the men in their lives to treat them as equals. She describes how women are subtly undermined in the home by men using disparaging stereotypes and being condescending. In the survey 70 per cent of women who had been married for more than five years said they were having extra-marital affairs, although almost all believed in monogamy and believed their husbands to be faithful. Ninety-one per cent of those who had divorced said that they made the decision to divorce, not their husbands – and not because of adultery or an unsatisfying sex life, but because of a sense of emotional isolation in the marriage.

In spite of greater permissiveness, then, all the evidence points to the relative rarity of female pleasure in sexual encounters. In view of the subordinate position of girls and the pervasiveness of sexual harassment, sex for girls can be a far from pleasant experience. Research into adolescent sexuality reflects the same dissatisfaction with sexual relationships.

How Possible is it to Change Sexual Practices?

The AIDS campaign has been aimed at altering the attitudes and sexual practices of young people to the use of condoms and other methods of birth-control. These studies generally find that knowledge of the risks of HIV infection is not a sufficient determinant of safe-sex practice. Information-giving is simply insufficient to bring about clear-cut and lasting behaviour changes. People actively 'make sense' of new ideas they encounter by assessing them in the light of pre-existing beliefs, interpreting them and fitting them in with their present knowledge (see Aggleton and Homans 1987). It is therefore essential to study the meanings attached to sexual relationships and how these change over time.

The reluctance of young people to alter their sexual behaviour has been well documented. According to a recent study involving interviews with young women, girls' identification as 'slags' or 'drags' is still prevalent, and current health-education programmes, based on increasing knowledge of condoms for protection against AIDS, overlook the meaning that the use of contraceptive technique has for young women and men and the ways in which their understanding differs (Holland et al. 1990).

Barbara Spencer (1984) held group discussions with adolescents aged between sixteen and nineteen from a variety of social backgrounds. The majority were comprised of boys only, but a few were mixed. A major finding was that there were striking differences between male and female views of sexual relations, with separate rules governing girls' and boys' behaviour. Only a third of sexually active teenagers used any contraception, which was more likely to be used in long term than casual relationships. Few boys saw themselves as respons-

ible for contraception, nor were they seen as responsible by
the girls. Spencer puts forward the following fascinating explanation which I discuss further in the chapter on violence:

The boys see their actions as governed by a set of social patterns
which are amoral and followed by almost all boys, whereas girls'
behaviour is seen as much less of a group phenomenon, with each
girl following her own personal moral code. This is compatible with
the general view that girls are consistently held responsible for their
actions, while boys are only expected to demonstrate responsibility
under certain conditions (Spencer 1984).

The low use of contraception by girls was partly explained
by girls' hesitancy about approaching doctors and birth-
control clinics, but what could be more significant is the
operation of the double standard that condemns a girl if she
plans to have sex. For young women to carry condoms around
implies premeditated sex, which conflicts with popular ideas of
romantic spontaneity and implicitly labels them as slags. The
operation of the double standard condemns a girl as irrespons-
ible if she does not use contraception and as unrespectable if
she does. If she uses contraception on a casual date this
contravenes the dominant code of romance, which opens her
up to savage criticism. To use contraception involves premedi-
tating sex, which is only legitimate with someone you are
'going steady' with. For a girl to have sex without contraception can only be explained as something which 'happens'
without previous intent unless of course the girl is a slag.

Some of the boys I interviewed thought that contraception
was a joint responsibility. Tony, an Italian boy, had listened
to his father's advice. When I asked him who should take
responsibility for contraception he replied:

Both, you discuss it beforehand. One, 'cos I don't have
a kid. 'Cos my dad told me there wasn't any contraception around in his day and he doesn't know how many
kids he has around Italy. And I got a message from that.

Jenny described when she went to a birth-control clinic

with her mother, who needed contraception. The woman at the clinic asked her if she wanted to go on the pill too. She refused but the woman said she might need to. Jenny replied:

> I've got will power. I didn't know what to say to her, I wouldn't go on it. I don't think it's right really because I know if you go on the pill you're going to lose will power in the end and just let yourself go.

Intriguingly, the phrase 'letting yourself go' has connections with both sexual excitement and becoming sluttish. Love seems to play an important ideological role in permitting the former while offering some protection from the latter.

On top of these considerations, condom use, unlike the pill, involves the boys' active collaboration and also requires a degree of confidence to handle. It involves talking about the sexual encounter rather than 'letting it happen', which is not only far more embarrassing to negotiate but also involves carrying condoms around with all the risks of exposure. A programme of sex education that would empower young women to take control of their own bodies to resist abuse and exploitation would be needed to begin to overcome these obstacles. Yet there is little sign that such action will be taken. For a woman to carry condoms can be seen as challenging the patriarchal definition of her as innately responsive to male initiative, as reactive rather than proactive. Such a challenge demands more than assertiveness training for women. It demands shifting the meaning of sexuality and of sexual identity (see Wilton and Aggleton 1990). The importance of a girl's self-esteem is crucial to her ability to insist on the use of condoms.

Generally surveys have found that young people are complacent about their risk of infection from HIV. Ford (1989b) in his study found only 30 per cent had used a condom in their last intercourse. Only one-fifth of the casual–recreational group who condoned sex outside a steady relationship used condoms. Abrams found that young people overestimate other people's involvement in casual sex. 'Most young people are adopting safe practices but, among the minority who are not, the key seems to be that they are unaware that they are in a minority. Their ignorance is not about the body. They cannot understand themselves because they do not know about other people's lives (Abrams 1991).

The Content of Sex Education

Critiques of the traditional nuclear family and the existing state of gender relations have hardly infiltrated the popular marriage literature or sex education in schools. In the USA sex education is also deficient. It has been estimated that as few as 2 per cent to 5 per cent of homes in the USA provide 'positive sex education' (Ramey 1980). Thornburg (1981) showed that among a large sample of teenagers from eleven different locations, young people estimated that they obtained about 40 per cent of all their information from their peers, and another 40 per cent from school literature. Only about 15 per cent was believed to come from parents. Mothers are more able to talk to their daughters than fathers to their sons. Sons are given little information. Tricia Szirom (1988), who carried out the most comprehensive study of sex-education provision undertaken in Australia, found that 60 per cent of young women chose their mother as their preferred person to learn about sex from, compared with 15 per cent of young men. Fathers were not a major source of information for either females or males. Some parents still do not provide even basic information, such as telling their daughters about periods. Brumberg (1992) reports a similar picture in the USA. Twenty-five per cent of questionnaire respondents who indicated that they could not talk to their parents about sex were more likely to have learned about sex from school or the media, with friends as a second source. A survey by *Seventeen* magazine in the USA, on the other hand, indicated that adolescents listed books and magazines as the second most common source of information, after their mothers (reported in Conger 1973).

Friends are a major source of misinformation according to a number of studies. A study conducted by Beighton et al. (1976) in Australia indicated that sources of formal information were useless and 84 per cent of the sample said friends were an informal source of information. Thomson and Scott (1991) found that the acquisition of knowledge from peers, particularly in the school context, is often a case of 'Chinese whispers'. Messages are progressively distorted as they circulate from person to person, obscuring sexual meanings that were not explicit to begin with. The young women we spoke to reported 'learning by "picking things up"' and 'just catching on'. Often this took the form of hearing sexual innuendo in the form of jokes, which, like 'reputation' can also serve the function of social censure. In Allen's (1987) sample, 30 per cent of teenagers thought that others of their age knew more about sex than themselves.

Most parents are in favour of school sex education. In 1984 in Canada a Gallup poll found that 83 per cent of parents were in favour of sex education in schools, though only 50 per cent of schools offered any (cited in Lenskyj 1990). Ninety-four per cent of British parents wish their children to receive sex education at school (Allen 1987). American parents feel the same; 98 per cent said they wanted help from the schools in talking to their teenage children about sex (Hudson and Ineichen 1991:179).

Recent findings in Britain concerning young people's sexual knowledge, attitudes and practices are no grounds for complacency. MORI interviewed a sample of 4,436 young people aged between sixteen and nineteen for the Health Education Authority, the results of which are assessed in the authority's Young Adults' Health and Lifestyle report published in August 1991. Most, 88 per cent, had received some sex education at school, though this varied in different parts of the country. Most sex education concentrated on how bodies develop, pregnancy and childbirth. Even the 'plumbing and prevention' focus was lacking, let alone discussion of such hazards as cervical cancer. Only two-thirds were taught about sexually transmitted diseases, only half about AIDS and a mere 14 per cent about lesbianism. An even larger gap concerned feeling and emotion, with only a third remembering being taught anything about them. Young people said they would like to have been taught about sexual relations and emotions, and more specifically about homosexuality and lesbianism. It is frequently assumed that people know a great deal about sexuality, sexual health, reproduction and contraception. This assumption is not borne out. They conclude that education about sexuality should include how to talk to each other.

There has been some improvement over the past ten years. A study of the attitudes of parents and fourteen- to sixteen-year-olds in three UK cities, one in the north-east, one in the Midlands and one in the south-west, carried out in the mid 1980s showed how far education in sex and personal relationships has come and the extent to which parents welcome the involvement of schools (see Allen 1987). However Thomson and Scott's 150 in-depth interviews with young women between the ages of sixteen and twenty-one in London and Manchester found the overall picture presented of school sex education was gloomy and it was given low priority within the curriculum, where sexual knowledge has often been seen as potentially dangerous. It was often subsumed into biology or hygiene classes. Training is badly needed (Thomson and Scott 1991).

A recent study of teenage pregnancy (Hudson and Ineichen 1991:36) found that the derogatory and censorious vocabulary used by boys and girls to describe girls' behaviour is a strong influence on the way girls see themselves. They too suggested that terms like 'slag' helped to keep a girl in her place and that girls who ended up as teenage mothers were often those who were caught up in a powerful web of sexual oppression. Getting pregnant was not simply due to ignorance but to girls adopting a 'it won't happen to me' attitude. They argued that surveys supported their findings that the majority of teenage pregnancies, even those carried to term, were initially unwanted events. Sharpe too found that few girls had deliberately set out to conceive.

The Politics and Provision of Sex Education

A number of studies have concluded that sex-education provision in Britain is still ad hoc and patchy (see Allen 1987, Thomson and Scott 1991). Attempts to provide services to young women, which might equip them to deal with changing realities, have included sex education in schools and greater availability of contraceptive advice and counselling. More recently this liberalization of sexual practices has been under attack in Britain from a Conservative government bent on reaffirming the virtues of premarital chastity and monogamy. In line with this, the Education Reform Act urges teachers to place sex education within the context of the morality of marriage and the family, and the 1988 Local Government Act outlaws the financing by local authorities of what is termed the 'promotion of homosexuality'. These two pieces of legislation have made it even more difficult for a broader approach to sexuality to be discussed in schools. In the USA too the far right is campaigning against abortion and 'attacks' on the family.

On the other hand, the recent legislation and guidance has for the first time provided a national framework for the provision of sex education for all pupils. The Education Reform Act 1988, by transferring the control of education from local education authorities to central government and school governing bodies, allows schools to 'opt out' of local authority control and manage their own finances. Responsibility for the organization of sex education in schools has also been transferred to governing bodies. Under the 1986 Education Act the governors of county and controlled schools were given a statutory obligation to decide whether sex education was to form part of the schools curriculum, and, if so, to draw up a written statement of their policy about its content and organization in the curriculum and to record that conclusion in writing (Department of Education and Science 1991). Furthermore it stated that the responsibility of every governing body should be 'to furnish the authority and the head teacher with an up to date copy of any statement (Education No. 2 Act 1986, section 18, 3c).

It is at present unclear how far these government interventions have affected the provision. The effectiveness varies from one part of the country to another. Sex education is reported as a disappointing source of information even when limited to providing adolescents with basic information about birth-control, sexually transmitted diseases and reproduction.

Responding to the widespread dissatisfaction with the provision among young people, in 1992 the Sex Education Forum, an umbrella body bringing together a range of organizations involved in supporting and advising on sex education to young people, conducted a survey of local education authority support for the monitoring of sex education (Thomson and Scott 1991). Levels of sex education were found to be very uneven. Where information was available the study found that 70 per cent of all schools had a written policy, 24 per cent had not yet developed a policy and 6 per cent had decided not to include sex education as part of the curriculum. In spite of the 1987 statutory obligation to develop a policy, a significant proportion still has not done so.

Implementation of Sex Education

Even when schools have developed policies, the implementation is often lacking for four reasons. Firstly, governors are often too over-committed to develop and monitor the implementation of policies. Secondly, the introduction of the national curriculum has meant there is little space for non-foundation subjects, particularly in secondary schools. There is some confusion concerning the place of sex education within the national curriculum, as some aspects are included in the statutory core subject of science, while other aspects are part of the non-statutory health education, which is given low priority. Thirdly, little training for teachers is provided. The Sex Education Forum survey encountered widespread anxiety at all levels concerned with the teaching of sex education. This anxiety was particularly acute in relation to fears of parental, governor and 'community' disapproval, as well as in relation to legislation. There is clearly an urgent need for training. The Sex Education Forum recommends that a specialist trained teacher should be present in each school who would coordinate all sex education and support other members of the sex-education team. Lastly, basic principles of implementing policies are rarely addressed.

The first problem of introducing sex education into schools is the difficulty girls and boys have of talking about the body and sexuality. For girls this is a greater problem than for boys. This is partly due to the lack of vocabulary and partly due to the contradictory way women's bodies, in particular, are viewed and how girls' identity and self-esteem are so closely contingent on their body image.

There is very little vocabulary to use to talk about the female sexual anatomy which is not derogatory or clinical. Carol Lee (1983) on setting up sex-education classes, met with opposition from head teachers over using certain words, such as vagina. Euphemisms for sex must be commoner in Britain than anywhere in the world: teachers are still censored for using words such as 'penetration' and many girls have no idea where to find their clitoris or vagina. Mothers are more reluctant to name the genital organs of their daughters than of their sons and tend to do so at a much later age. Many mothers are embarrassed to name the girl's sexual organs at all except by referring to her 'bottom'. The only word the girl may come into contact with is 'cunt', which is depicted as dirty and shameful. There are no acceptable words for female sexual parts, though 'fanny' is perhaps one possibility. Most social stereotypes define women's genitals as unpleasant, odorous and unattractive and these stereotypes are internalized by the female child. Many of the obscenities directed at women are so taken for granted that girls and women stop noticing them.

> If they're all girls and the boys aren't here, we can talk
> to the teacher about the facts of life and growing up and
> abortion and things like that (Jane, aged fifteen).

A girl finds talking about sexuality and the body difficult for the very reason that her body is so much linked to her identity.

Depictions of a girl's body are the raw material of sexist abuse. At the same time her appearance is presented as her passport to success both in private and public life. One of the strongest bases of self-esteem rests on pride in body image. The widespread dissatisfaction that girls express about their physical attractiveness is startling. Not one girl expressed pride and confidence in good looks. Anxiety often focuses on their bodies. Adolescent girls are more likely than boys to report that they have difficulty in adjusting to their changed body images between the ages of twelve and sixteen. Research indicates that girls are more likely to experience depersonalization because their self-concepts are much more volatile at this age. Germaine Greer found that the young themselves are unaware of their bloom, and deeply insecure about their attractiveness (Greer 1991). It is clear that girls' bodies are subject to contradictory appraisal. A girl is constantly warned that her body may let her down, by emitting unpleasant odours or leaking. Menstruation is a constant concern. As Germaine Greer comments:

One of the first skills a young woman has to develop is that of dealing with menstruation in mixed company without anybody guessing what they are about, slipping into the lavatory with a sanitary napkin up a sleeve, washing stained underwear on the sly in co-ed digs. It is arguable that young women would find menstruation less problematic if they did not have to behave as if they were ashamed of it (Greer 1991).

Wood (1984:65) in his study of a small unit for disruptive adolescents describes how 'the reproductive and excremental aspects of the female body were constantly referred to by the boys in that fixated, disgusted tone, edged with nervousness and surrounded by giggling'. He points out that there is no equivalent way girls discuss boys' bodies and that it appeared to him that 'women as a whole are sometimes regarded by men as dirty, alien, even evil'. Paul Willis (1977) in his study of working-class lads carried out in the late 1970s also portrayed many of their views as blatantly sexist, exemplified by their fascination with 'jam rags' (sanitary towels). Boys in both these studies talk endlessly about bodies in relation to sex and sexual pleasure but are quite unable to deal with childbirth, breast-feeding or the logistics of contraception. Our culture reinforces this. Women are ostracized for feeding a baby in a restaurant. This represents a disgust with the female body when it is being treated apart from reference to male sexual pleasure.

The stereotype to emulate is of a thin Linda Evangelista or Naomi Campbell, a model where thinness is elevated to the highest moral plane. Over and over again in my interviews girls expressed a wish to be different. Usually this involved a desire to be slim, but when a girl was slim, she still did not see herself as attractive. Amy, an Asian girl, sighs:

I wish I had a different body.
Q *What do you mean?*
A bit fatter. I think I am too skinny.
Q *Do you admire other girls' bodies?*
I think there is always something wrong with a girl's body. There is always something wrong. They're not perfect. I've always got that in mind. They've never got the right figure.
Q *What is the right figure?*

> Don't know. Not the right figure, you know, um, not too
> skinny not too fat. Just medium height. 5 foot 7 inches,
> 26-inch waist. Nice long hair, and nice all the rest.

Faced with these contradictions, some girls use avoidance
tactics, relinquish all desire and stay away from boys, sex and
even food. Anxiety often focuses on their bodies. Anorexia and
bulimia among privileged white adolescent girls have reached
'epidemic' proportions according to some American sources
(see Brumberg 1992). The increasing prevalence of such eating
disorders among female adolescents can be understood as a
way of girls' clutching on to an identity that is experienced as
disintegrating. A split between the body and self can occur
where the only way the girl can regain control is to starve (see
Orbach 1986). For some girls anorexia is mild and transitory,
others, perhaps as many as 19 per cent of diagnosed cases, die
from it (Halmi et al. 1975). Yet all girls are affected by what
Naomi Wolf has called 'the beauty myth'. No wonder that all
my daughter's adolescent friends consider that they are too fat
and are dissatisfied with their appearance. Or, as we shall see
in Chapter 7, girls develop tactics of resistance, some more
successful than others. In explaining the taboo on menstruation, Sophie Laws (1990), who undertook an in-depth study of
men's attitudes to menstruation, argues that these taboos are
inseparable from how men see women generally. Viewing
menstruation so negatively makes it difficult for women to talk
about it and to feel positive about themselves. Male culture
portrays men as absolutely in control of sex with women,
rendering menstruation threatening, since it has nothing to do
with men or sex.

Male joking attempts to bring menstruation under male
control, as it perhaps unconsciously reminds them of their own
humanity (that they were born) and has an association with
'nature', from which maleness attempts so hard to dissociate
itself. Male joking can be seen as the remnants of the menstruation rituals which prescribed women to be kept separate
during their periods. Male unease with discussing anything

relating to childbirth, menopause, contraception or even their own bodies derives from this discourse of masculinity that denies their biological heritage and their dependence on women.

Female sexual experience is constructed in terms of male action, and girls have no vocabulary or language in which to formulate their sexual experience, the very expression of which threatens their social standing. All this adds up to the need for the suppression of sexual desire. And of course the boys are disadvantaged too. They may be 'dominant', but the pressure towards hegemonic masculinity can only lead them to suppress their sensitivity and feelings of vulnerability that then emerge in brutality and fights. The practices are just as powerful in constructing male sexuality.

Secondly, little thought is given to how sex education should be introduced to different groups, of different racial backgrounds and of different gender. Amrit Wilson found that the issue of sex education brought Asian girls into conflict between school and home values. Many Asian parents, whether Hindu, Muslim or Sikh, were against the idea of sex education (Wilson 1978). The Sex Education Forum took the view that the development of sex-education policies may be avoided because of assumptions of parental and community opposition which they consider may be based on stereotypical views both of the attitudes of communities and of the nature of sex education. However, it is more likely that there are some real conflicts between the aims of a liberal sex-education policy and some religious groups. The need for adequate training so that conflicts can be understood and dealt with sensitively is clearly very important.

What topics should be raised in single-sex groups, and what topics in mixed groups is another important issue. Sex education is usually taught in mixed groups, although there are strong arguments for topics such as menstruation and childbirth to be raised in single-sex groupings. One of the few studies to examine in detail the way one school (a large East

Midlands comprehensive) handles sex-education classes found that although teachers are well meaning and spend an inordinate time planning the classes, the gap between the sessions and the adolescents' sexual world is enormous (see Measor 1989). A group of twelve-year-olds reacted with great embarrassment to mixed sex-education classes particularly when taken by a male teacher. When watching a film on reproduction and birth, the boys nudged each other and giggled and the atmosphere was uncomfortable. In some schools the discussion of menstruation has taken place in mixed groups, on the grounds that this will break any taboos about openness. This seems a very naïve assumption. In the Policy Studies Unit study half the girls said they found single-sex groups were less embarrassing, but more boys preferred mixed groups. There is a strong case for single-sex groups, though it may be appropriate to discuss issues such as abortion and parenting in mixed groups. Discussion in single-sex groups could perhaps also be followed by mixed-sex discussions. The Sex Education Forum survey found that only ten local education authorities monitored gender grouping in mixed schools. Seven of these were of the view that while occasional segregation was useful for a specific aspect, teaching should otherwise be in normal teaching groups. Two proposed all mixed teaching and one left it to schools to decide. Only one suggested that 'valuable work can be done in girls' groups in developing self-esteem' (Thomson and Scott 1991).

To show sensitive and highly explicit films on giving birth is quite inappropriate in mixed groups. Several of the adolescent girls I interviewed who viewed a film about birth in a mixed group experienced great embarrassment. The lack of imagination in showing films in this way illustrates Measor's point about the gap between the two worlds of teachers and adolescents. Girls were upset by the depiction of so many more naked female bodies than male. It is likely this embarrassment is due to the way they are bombarded by such depictions in advertisements, films and newspapers outside school. This

may be one reason why some girls do not think it appropriate
to discuss sex in school. Portraying nudity has a different
meaning for men and women. Men's nudity is not part of
everyday life and does not denote sexual provocativeness in
the same way as female nudity.

> When we talk about childbirth in school boys go all
> stupid ... Like we saw a film the other day with a lady
> having a baby and the boys were just so stupid. The girls
> were really sensible, just watching and the boys were
> getting all carried away, all worked up about it ... The
> teacher goes, 'I'm ashamed of you.' She thought they
> would have been old enough to know how a lady has a
> baby and that. She was really ashamed of the boys 'cos
> we were with another class. Her class, I think. The boys
> were laughing and shouting things over to the girls ...
> being stupid.

From a young age girls are presented with images of the
female body but at the same time taught to cover themselves up, sit demurely with their legs together and be
discreet. No wonder that sex-education classes cause
embarrassment.

Teachers too are often embarrassed to talk about sexual
issues. There is an even greater reluctance to challenge sexism.
Both these issues need to be addressed. Even men who are
relatively enlightened regarding sexism rarely contest it, perhaps in dread of being considered 'wimpish'. Few feel able to
question boys' sexism, let alone the sexism of their colleagues.
As two researchers commented on the difficulty of introducing
anti-sexist initiatives into schools:

The male teachers did not feel able, within the confines of the school,
actively to challenge and question boys' assumptions ... Whilst
feminist teachers are actively challenging and confronting pupils
regarding their sexist prejudices all the time. It has to be said that
the reluctance of men teachers to do the same inhibits the process of
change and, on educational grounds, is insufficient (Cornbleet and
Sanders 1982).

In some London schools attempts are being made to encourage teachers to contest sexism as well as racism. Tony is more sympathetic to contesting racist terms, but is aware that sexist language is also an issue:

> In this school teachers tell you off if you use sexist language. Not every teacher, but most. But we have more discussion about racism and racist terms. That's something I'm more against.

Yet the sexism rampant in many schools needs to be seriously challenged. Boys at adolescence suddenly start to describe girls in terms of their body parts. A dissecting approach is often taken to women's objectified bodies. As Julian Wood points out, in many of the discussions that men hold on the subject of women, the assumption is that a woman can be assessed solely in terms of male opinion of parts of the female body – arse, 'boat', legs and so on. To consider each and every woman only from the point of view of conquest, to describe women via parts of their bodies – face, tits, ginger minge (pubic hair) – is a reflection of the sexist ways women are depicted in advertisements and popular culture. 'Extrapolating from this attitude I think it is not too fanciful to say that women as a whole are sometimes regarded by men as dirty, alien, even evil' (Wood 1984:65).

In his study of British boys attending a youth club in the early 1980s, he gives an example of a boy indulging in this favourite pastime by cataloguing the qualities of a friend's sister. The boy is trying to persuade his friend that the girl is attractive: 'She's lovely, ginger minge, oh my good God! You don't fuck the face and she's got a nice body, so what are you worried about?' The assumption is that a 'nice body' can be traded against a presumably bad face. Julian Wood does not express sufficient horror that boys should describe a girl in this appalling way or explain why such misogynism flourishes.

Mary Daly calls this male talk 'spooking from the locker room':

Most of the time the language is used in all male environments. Yet it is the common male view of all women and, although most women do not hear it directly, we receive the message in a muted way. It is conveyed through silences, sneers, jeers, excessive politeness, paternalistic praise and disapproval, aggressive physical contact, an arm around the shoulder, a pat on the behind, invasive stares. Since women often do not hear the messages of obscenity directly, we are spooked. For the invasive presence and the intent are both audible and inaudible, visible and invisible. Moreover, women are conditioned to pretend not to hear/see the constant and violent bombardments of obscenity, for we have been taught the lesson that since verbal violence is a 'substitute' for physical assault, we should be grateful for such seemingly mild manifestations of misogyny. Thus, spooking from the locker room, the unacknowledged noise of omnipresent male obscenities, constitutes the 'background music' which continually confuses and fragments consciousness. Exorcizing this invasive presence requires acknowledging its existence and refusing to shuffle. This has the effect of bringing the spookers out into the open (Daly 1978:323).

The taboo surrounding menstruation is another issue that needs to be challenged. Sophie Laws asked a group of men about menstruation and found that men used quite distinctive terms, quite separate vocabularies, about menstruation from women, most of them derogatory. She discovered that half in her sample reported boys joking about menstruation. The most common term used was 'jam rag' (and its variants, jam sandwich, jam roll) for sanitary towel. Boys would put girls down with phrases such as, 'She's on', to denote that a girl was ruled by her hormones. Men also reported boys making dirty jokes about menstruation between themselves. One man even reported the term 'jam rag' being used by a boy to put another boy down. More than half the adult men had also heard jokes about menstruation. Most of these jokes quite explicitly portrayed women as sex objects and as interchangeable. So, as one man said: 'You used to say "Oh hard luck" kind of thing [*laughs*] picking the wrong one' (Laws 1990:47).

Virginia Ernster in her article 'American Menstrual

Euphemisms' also found two different sets of terms used by men and women, the ones men used having sexual and derogatory connotations, the ones women used partly having the function of communicating to other women their condition without men realizing it. The case for single-sex groupings to discuss menstruation seems irrefutable. In Britain there have been some experiments in mixed schools with single-sex classes, the establishment of girls-only groups and support groups for women teachers. Without single-sex groupings, sex education can be counterproductive and girls can be the scapegoats of boys' unease. Mixed groups can promote rather than dispel prejudices.

Sex education can support rather than challenge the dominant sexism in society. Sex education is not politically neutral. Three political stances can be differentiated.

The Conservative Stance

Sex education has always been an area of controversy, which explodes periodically in panic about the so-called decline of real values and the breakdown of the family. The move to the right in America and parts of Europe bears a frightening resemblance to the right-wing ideology of the McCarthy period in America. There non-familial sex was linked with communism and political weakness. During this period Kinsey and the Institute of Sex Research were attacked for weakening the moral fibre of Americans and rendering them vulnerable to communist influence. In 1969 the extreme right discovered the Sex Information and Education Council (SIECUS) and attacked sex education as a communist plot to destroy the family and sap national will. Sex education was attacked in books and pamphlets such as *The Sex Education Racket: Pornography in the Schools* and *SIECUS: Corrupter of Youth* (Rubin 1984:173).

The New Right and new conservative ideology in the USA has updated these links between immoral sexual behaviour and the decline of American power. In 1977 Norman

Podhoretz blamed homosexuals for the alleged inability of the USA to stand up to the Soviets. Right-wing fundamentalist religious crusaders are against abortion, premarital sex and homosexuality. As the recession deepens equal rights legislation has been defeated and access to abortion is becoming more restricted. The 1973 *Roe v. Wade* decision where the Supreme Court found abortion to be a matter of privacy between a woman and her doctor has been challenged though not reversed. Organizations such as the Moral Majority and Citizens for Democracy have acquired mass followings. The Family Protection Act introduced into Congress in 1979 was an assault on feminism, homosexuals, on non-traditional families and teenage sexual privacy. Fifteen million dollars was allocated to a Teen Chastity program to encourage teenagers to refrain from sexual intercourse (Rubin 1984:274). In Britain too during the last few years the soaring divorce rate, the spread of AIDS, the rise in single-parent families and increasing 'permissiveness' is thought by the right to be evidence of the moral decline of the nation.

Education is seen as one means of resisting this decline. The conservative view stresses that sex education should be concerned with the preservation of the family and the preparation of young men and women to fulfil their roles. In Britain in many schools little has changed in sex education from the Church of England Board of Education 1962 specifications that in sex education the emphasis should be on preparation for marriage and that physical, spiritual and moral elements should be included, with great emphasis laid on the traditional family. In this model sex is equated with marriage for girls. Teaching is predominantly concerned with the suppression of sex outside marriage, with the physical aspects of reproduction within marriage and with what has been defined as the abnormal, which in males takes the form of VD and in females illegitimate births or pregnancies (see Wolpe 1988: 104).

Viscount Buckmaster, who presented the new amendment

to the Education Bill to the House of Lords, claimed 'The image that we want to promote in our schools is one of family life based on stable, loving, and adaptive relationships and of the family as a life-giving unit, and not some of the modern variants which are accepted on occasions' (Hansard, 2 June 1986).

This view fails to take into account that marriage holds many advantages for young men, but young women are beginning to demand a great deal more from their partners than previously. According to Szirom's study (1988) in Australia, while young men are still expressing traditional attitudes, many women have a sophisticated analysis of the nature of relationships between the sexes – and they don't like what they see. This is why marriage has recently become less popular. Feminists such as Dinnerstein and Chodorow argue that until men take part more fully in bringing up children, the misogyny of present-day society will remain unchanged. Sex education should ideally involve courses on child development and education for shared parenting.

The Liberal Stance

The liberal approach to sex education is concerned mainly with providing children with information so that they are able to make informed choices. However, the information at present provided is often very limited and takes little account of the context of sexual relationships. It is too often centred on the preparation for the traditional family. Ann Marie Wolpe, for example, who carried out research in a mixed Greater London secondary school found that the Local Education Adviser, a Miss Jack, advised parents at a parents' meeting that her lessons would deal with sources of infection, changes in the child's pituitary gland (which is directly related to the process of reproduction), the menstrual cycle and puberty and, finally, childcare and nutrition. She was opposed to dealing with questions of human relationships until children were much older. Childcare did not question woman's role in the family.

Privately she commented, 'What I really think sex education is all about is to get the boys and girls to play their correct roles.' Sexual relationships were only referred to obliquely and only in the context of monogamous marriage. Any consideration involving emotional relationships could not be included within a school curriculum directly.

In Australia approximately half of the sex-education programmes in schools are science- or biology-based and reproduction is the topic most often covered. Szirom (1988) reports that students complain that they are not given the opportunity to discuss the implications of human relationships, issues involved in such things as contraception, abortion or the problems they have in communication and forming relationships.

The way sex education is taught has not significantly changed over the years from this 'plumbing and prevention' focus. The HMI discussion document, 'Health Education from 5–16', stipulated that when taught in primary schools sex education should be 'presented in the context of family life, of loving relationships and of respect for others: in short in a moral framework' (p. 5).

The Feminist Stance

A feminist approach to sex education would be aimed at challenging the sexism that is so taken for granted by boys and girls. Both in method and content it would have a very different focus from present teaching, which is constructed on a male view of sexuality. The sexual revolution of the 1970s undoubtedly opened up discussion about sexuality, but has done little to affect the balance of power in heterosexual relationships. Constructs of masculinity and femininity would be challenged.

This new approach would focus on the moral dilemmas of living, the importance of relationships for both boys and girls and equal responsibility in relationships.

To understand the representation of female sexuality, it is useful to consider what defines male sexuality. Litewka (1977) suggests that the main aim of male sexuality is penile penetration and ejaculation. This process requires, according to Litewka, first objectification, making women into 'a concept, a lump sum, a thing, an object, a non-individualized category', then fixation on 'portions of the female anatomy' to make her even more distant and unreal, and finally conquest. He comments that the sexual level is the only level at which he could not accept women as equals. For women and men to make love equally involves divesting oneself of the construction of masculinity as dominant and necessarily penetrative.

Such an approach is outlined by Tricia Szirom, who draws on her wide experience as education director of the Family Planning Association of Victoria, Australia. She argues the preventative approach, emphasizing birth-control, reproduction and VD, epitomized a male approach to sex education, not at all geared towards young women who had different needs. Young men's traditional attitudes to sex should be questioned and links between sexism and sex education drawn. From her research she concludes that students are not assisted to explore the assumptions about male sexuality within the broader culture, nor to value female sexuality other than as a reproductive function.

She demonstrates that schools are constructing a male view of sexuality, both in the content of sex-education programmes and the classroom practice used to present materials. Her research shows that by providing sex education in mixed-sex classes, by allowing, yet again, the males to define the content of programmes and by the very language and focus of such programmes, a biased view of sexuality for both females and males is constructed. Schools replicate sexist attitudes and stereotypes, thus adding to the disadvantages experienced by girls and women in their relationships with males. She concludes: 'Sexuality programmes in schools should address directly the underlying attitudes and socialization forces that discriminate against women who make their own choices and equip young men to become full and equal partners in this important aspect of their lives' (Szirom 1988:139).

Philip Meredith (1989) argues that we could learn a great deal from the Swedish sex-education system, where curricular guidelines have been agreed by consultation. Sweden is the first country in the world to have established an official sex-education curriculum for schools which is compulsory. Contraception and human relationships are dealt with in depth. The general goals set out include the phrase 'responsibility, consideration and care for their fellow beings, and in this way experiencing sexuality as a source of happiness together with another person'. This emphasis, rather than the usual stress on risk, disease and moral degradation, gives the Swedish system a ground of humanity.

Questions such as what should be taught, what degree of teacher autonomy is appropriate, and whose values should sex education reflect are on the agenda. The limitation of aims in the USA and Britain needs to be questioned. In the USA the need for relationship education is gradually being recognized. Planned Parenthood programs are being introduced combined with education and, in some states (for example in Minnesota), teenage pregnancies have dramatically dropped (Hudson and Ineichen 1991:180).

Progressive Attempts

In some schools progressive approaches to sex education have resulted in a storm of controversy. In 1983 a little-known book, *Jenny Lives with Eric and Martin*, dealing with the life of a young girl living with her gay father and his lover, generated a storm of anti-gay publicity. Such initiatives have been seen by some as a direct attack on the family. In October 1986 the *London Standard* (22 October 1986) front page blazed BEWARE THIS DIRTY DOZEN. Peter Bruinvels, an MP and a member of the Family Campaign drew up a list of thirteen books which were then nicknamed 'Baker's dozen'. These included *Make it Happy* by Jane Cousins, the British Medical Association's *Sex for Beginners*, *Talking Sex* by Miriam Stoppard and the above-mentioned book about two homosexuals raising a child.

Bruinvels led a backbench revolt over government plans for sex education, campaigning for the right of parents to with-draw their children from classes, and for new powers to enable the Education Secretary to ban books and sack teachers who use such books (Langford and Pfeffercorn 1988). Women MPs were attacked: Emma Nicholson, the Conservative MP for Devon West and Torridge, recalls a debate on abortion when a Labour woman's description of the suffering that back-street abortions caused was greeted with taunts from Conservative backbenchers of 'She's a slut. She's a slag. She's had enough of them so she should know' (Nadel 1990). AIDS fuelled even greater anti-gay publicity, culminating in the notorious Clause 28 of the Local Government Act of 1988, which forbids councils to 'intentionally promote homosexuality'.

Sex education rarely raises issues of sexual orientation. In some schools in the last five years a few attempts have been made to go much further with the aim of helping students to understand and accept their differences in sexual orientation. In these schools homosexuality has been presented as a valid lifestyle and the idea of a single, morally correct norm is discouraged. This more radical approach to sex education involving the questioning of heterosexism and the double standard of sexual morality has met with considerable resist-ance, though some teachers quietly broadened sex education to include real issues facing young people, including questions of sexual orientation.

Pat Mahony (1992), a British feminist educationalist, de-scribes how some teachers have managed to keep equal opportunities criteria at the forefront of the restructuring of education in drawing up the new curriculum. They have used the government's documentation to their own advantage by finding 'hooks' to hang their equal opportunity 'hats' on. She illustrates how there is still room to develop feminist approaches with the introduction of the national curriculum in state schools. In each subject the first task would be to identify major aims, such as enabling girls to grasp the mechanisms of male dominance and the strategies women have used past and present to resist such domination. She sees the introduction of the national curriculum as an opportunity to achieve our aims and identify major questions:

These might include asking, How well do we enable girls to achieve economic independence? How far does school operate with preconceptions about what constitutes appropriate work for white middle-class girls or working-class Asian girls (or vice versa)? How can we enable them to grasp the varieties of male violence, and how can we foster a culture in the school where their sense of self-worth is such that they grow up believing in their own dignity as human beings? How can they come to value the diversity of female strength and how can we affirm and radicalize what traditionally have been regarded as female skills?

She suggests that in looking at the question of sports, the question of which sports are played by women or men and why, and comparing different countries, English may be used to establish the role of language in reflecting, maintaining and reconstituting oppression, while modern languages can reinforce the point by illustrating and consolidating it. Or again, in personal, social and health education we can directly explore the ways social divisions are maintained, and science can follow this up by including under the unit of energy questions such as 'Why has solar energy not been more highly developed? Who benefits?'

Sexual harassment and violence are other areas that badly need to be addressed in school sex education. The way that violence is condoned will be taken up in the next chapter.

My research can be seen as uncovering the way that boys have power over girls to dominate and oppress. Gender dominance is institutionalized within practices of school, the language, the culture and our social and legal institutions, which makes it very difficult to resist. The questioning of 'taken for granted' practices of everyday life is an essential first step to introducing sex education into schools. In the next chapter I shall explore the problem of violence and sexual harassment in schools, which should also be part of any sex-education programme.

Notes

1. The denial of the whole person in school was dramatically illustrated by the treatment of Lisa Nussbaum, who appeared at school with bruises on her face several days before being murdered by her stepfather, an eminent New York lawyer. The school photographer noticed the bruises and told her to move so that the bruises would not be visible in the class photograph. Teachers presumably ignored the bruising too.

Bibliography

Abrams, D., 1991, *Aids: What Young People Believe and What They Do*, University of Kent

Aggleton, P., and Homans, A., 1987, *Education in Sex and Personal Relationships*, Policy Studies Institute

Allen, I., 1987, *Education in Sex and Personal Relationships*, Policy Study Institute Research Report No. 665

Beighton, F., Cole, J., and Howard, D., 1976, Submission to the Royal Commission on Human Relationships, University of Melbourne, quoted in Szirom, 1988

British Youth Council, 1992, *The Time of Your Life? The Truth About Being Young in '90s Britain*

Brumberg, J., 1992, 'Something Happens to Girls; The Changing Experience of Menarche in American Girls', paper given at the Alice in Wonderland Conference, Amsterdam, June 1992

Bury, J., 1984, *Teenage Pregnancy in Britain*, Birth Control Trust

Chalker, R., and Downer, C., *A Woman's Book of Choices: Abortion, Menstrual Extraction, RU-486*, Four Walls Eight Windows

Conger, J., 1973, *Adolescence and Youth*, Harper and Row

Conger, J., and Petersen, A., 1984, *Adolescence and Youth*, Harper and Row

Cornbleet, A., and Sanders, S., 1982, *Designing Anti-sexist Initiatives*, Inner London Education Authority

Daly, M., 1978, *Gyn/Ecology: The Metaphysics of Radical Feminism*, Beacon Books

Department of Education and Science, 1991, briefing document, 'The School Curriculum'

Ernster, V., 1975, 'American Menstrual Euphemisms', *Sex Roles*, 1, 1

Estaugh, V., and Wheatley, J., 1990, 'Family Planning and Family Well Being', Occasional Paper No. 12, London Family Policy Studies Centre

Farrell, C., 1978, *My Mother Said: The Way Young People Learned About Sex*, Routledge and Kegan Paul

Ford, N., 1989, 'Urban-rural Variations in the Level of Heterosexual Activity of Young People', in *Area*, 21.3, pp. 237–248

Ford, N., 1991, 'The Socio-sexual Lifestyles of Young People in South-west England', South-western Regional Health Authority Institute of Population Studies

Ford, N., and Morgan, 1989, 'Heterosexual Lifestyles of Young People in an English City', in *Journal of Population and Social Studies*, Vol. 1, No. 2, Jan.

Francome, C., 1986, *Abortion Practice in Britain and the United States*, Allen and Unwin

Fuller, M., 1980, 'Black Girls in a London Comprehensive School', in Deem, R. (ed.), *Schooling for Women's Work*, Routledge and Kegan Paul

Greer, G., 1991, *The Change*, Hamish Hamilton

Halmi, K., Broadland, G., and Rigas, C., 1975, 'A Follow-up Study of 79 Patients with Anorexia Nervosa: An Evaluation of Prognostic Factors and Diagnostic Criteria', in *Life History Research in Psychopathology*, Wirt, R.D., Winokur, G., and Roff, M. (eds.), Vol. 4

Hauer, L. B., 1989, 'Pregnancy and HIV Infection', *Focus: A Guide to AIDS Research* 4 (11), pp. 1–2

Hite, S., 1976, *The Hite Report: A Nationwide Study of Sexuality*, Macmillan

Hite, S., 1988, *Women and Love: A Cultural Revolution in Progress*, Knopf

HMSO, 1990, Social Trends, Tables 1.12 and 2.26

HMSO, 1992, 'The Health of the Nation: A Strategy for Health in England', p. 99

Holland, J., Ramazanoglu, C., and Scott, S., 1990, 'Managing Risk and Experiencing Danger: Tensions between government

AIDS-education policy and young women's sexuality', *Gender and Education*, Vol. 2, No. 2

Hudson, F., and Ineichen, B., 1991, *Taking it Lying Down: Sexuality and Teenage Motherhood*, Macmillan

Langford, D., and Pfeffercorn, A., 1988, 'Sex Education: Who Needs It?', *GEN* Challenging Heterosexism March

Laws, S., 1991, 'Issues of Blood', *Trouble and Strife*, 20, Spring

Lee, C., 1983, *The Ostrich Position*, Writers and Readers Lesbian and Gay Youth

Lenskyj, H., 1990, 'Beyond Plumbing and Prevention: Feminist Approaches to Sex Education', in *Gender and Education*, Vol. 2, No. 2

Lesbian and Gay Rights, Coalition for, 1988, report on high school, quoted in Lenskyj, H., Beyond Plumbing and Prevention: Feminist Approaches to Sex Education', *Gender and Education*, Vol. 2, No. 2

Litewka, J., 1977, 'The Socialized Penis', in Snodgrass, J. (ed.), *A Book of Readings for Men Against Sexism*, Times Change Press

Mahony, P., 1992, 'Which Way Forward? Equality and Schools in the 1990s', in *Women's Studies International Forum*, Vol. 15, No. 2

McRobbie, A., 1991, *Feminism and Youth Culture: From 'Jackie' to 'Just Seventeen'*, Macmillan

Measor, L., 1989, 'Are you coming to see some dirty films today?', in Holly, L. (ed.), 'Sex Education and Adolescent Sexuality', in *Girls and Sexuality*, Open University Press

Meredith, P., 1989, *Sex Education: Political Issues in Britain and Europe*, Routledge and Kegan Paul

Nadel, J., 1990, 'Male Chauvinist MPs', in the *Guardian*, 18 July 1990

Orbach, S., 1986, *Fat is a Feminist Issue*, Arrow

Patton, C., and Kelly, J., 1987, *Making It: A Woman's Guide to Sex in the Age of AIDS*, Firebrand

Ramey, J., 1980, Lecture at the Royal Children's Hospital, Melbourne, May 1980, quoted in Szirom 146:10

Rich, A., 1980, *Against Compulsory Heterosexuality*, Onlywoman Press

Richardson, D., 1987, *Women and the AIDS Crisis* (2nd edition), Pandora

Rubin, G., 1984, 'Thinking Sex', in Vance, C. (ed.), *Pleasure and Danger*, Routledge and Kegan Paul

Sex Education Forum, 1992, *A Framework for School Sex Education*

Sharpe, S., 1987, *Falling for Love*, Virago

Spencer, B., 1984, 'Young Men: Their Attitudes Towards Sexuality and Birth Control', *British Journal of Family Planning*, 10:13–19, p. 14

Squirrell, G., 1989, 'Teachers and Issues of Sexual Orientation', in *Gender and Education*, Vol. 1, No. 1

Szirom, P., 1988, *Teaching Gender*, Allen and Unwin

Thomson, R., and Scott, S., 1991, 'Learning About Sex: Young Women and the Social Construction of Sexual Identity', WRAP Paper 4, Tufnell Park Press

Thornburg, H. D., 1981, 'Adolescent Sources of Information on Sex', in *Journal of Social Health*, April 1981, pp. 274–7

Trenchard, L., and Warren, H., 1984, *Something to Tell You*, London Gay Teenage Group

Vinovskis, M., 1988, *An epidemic of Teenage Pregnancy? Some historical and policy considerations*, Oxford University Press

Voydanoff, P., and Donnelly, B., 1990, 'Adolescent Sexuality and Pregnancy', in *Family Studies Text*, Series 12, Sage Publications

Willis, P., 1977, *Learning to Labour*, Saxon House

Wilson, A., 1978, *Finding a Voice*, Virago

Wilton, T., and Aggleton, P., 1990, 'Young People and Safer Sex', paper given at the First Scandinavian Conference on Safer Sex, Stockholm

Wolpe, A. M., 1988, *Within School Walls: The Role of Discipline, Sexuality and the Curriculum*, Routledge and Kegan Paul

Wood, J., 1984, 'Groping Towards Sexism: Boys' Sex Talk', in McRobbie, A., and Nava, M. (eds.), *Gender and Generation*, Macmillan

Zelnick, M., and Kantner, J. F., 1980, 'Sexual Activity, Contraceptive Use and Pregnancy Among Metropolitan Area Teenagers: 1971–1979', *Family Planning Perspectives*, 12, pp. 230–37

Chapter 6

Violence and Bullying

Violence and bullying of girls at school is becoming a more recognized problem (see Mahony 1985), but few policies have been developed to deal with it effectively. The male aggression that pervades many classrooms and playgrounds, often undetected by teachers and parents, is, if not a direct consequence, certainly linked to the way violence is constituted as an important facet of masculinity. Violence and bullying do not take place in a vacuum, nor are they unambiguously biologically determined. Male violence is condoned, female anger outlawed. Aggression is a central attribute of masculinity and in a culture where male status is dependent on superiority and dominance, fighting prowess is crucial to that status. Manual work, even in the form of 'dead-end jobs', as Paul Willis showed, is another source of male status, which is why his working-class lads embraced them. But now many working-class boys are facing unemployment and can no longer gain a masculine identity through work. Other sources of masculine status, sexual prowess, joy-riding and fighting to obtain status in same-sex groups, at least as far as working-class boys are concerned, have become even more important and unless alternative models of masculinity are adopted, violence against women and between men is likely to increase.

Girls can be bullies too and sometimes fight each other, as we shall see in the next chapter, but overt aggression is relatively rare precisely because girls are discouraged from expressing anger. More commonly girls' anger, along with their active sexuality, is suppressed. Anger may be displaced or turned inwards to emerge as drug abuse, bodily disorders, anorexia and bulimia or depression. Bullying of girls often takes the form of attacks on a girl's sexual reputation and can lead to low self-esteem. The way that femininity is constituted in early childhood, when parents inadvertently discourage the expression of anger in their daughters and encourage it in their sons, contributes to very different rates of aggression among girls and boys in later life.

In this chapter the relation between the attitudes of both girls and boys to male violence will be analysed. Intrinsic to this is our society's ambivalent and contradictory attitude to male sexuality and aggression.

Attitudes to Violence

Research on violent behaviour is prolific, but little is known about sex differences in attitudes to violence or how sex differences in socialization can lead to the approval of violence. Views of violence are contradictory: it is both condoned and deplored. An American study shows that the majority of their respondents approve of violence when it is a means to a desired end. A constellation of values corresponding to traditional masculine values – bravery, retributive justice and physical ability to defend oneself and win – are associated with greater approval of violence. These values can be seen as a central component of American culture (see Blumenthal et al. 1972) but they can also been seen as central components of masculinity.

Often the responsibility for arousing aggression is subtly shifted on to girls. It is widely believed, for example, that male sexual drives, once aroused, are uncontrollable, and the arousal results from girls' so-called provocative behaviour. Wearing a short skirt was considered sufficient provocation not long ago, but with girls now donning hot-pants, and skirts shortening to the thighs, flaunting sexuality in girls is encouraged by the fashion industry. In spite of this there is an ambivalence in attitudes to young women, depicted in rape trials where the clothing of the woman complainant is still considered relevant to whether or not the defendant was led on (see Lees 1989a and b). The dominant form of masculinity encourages boys to pressure girls into sex. This is rationalized as a natural assertion of maleness, rather than a means of confirming male status. But to behave in this way involves objectifying women, denying their subjectivity, rejecting reciprocity. Girls too condone male violence and sometimes condemn other girls for reputed sexual promiscuity. Bullying and fighting among girls is often incited by attacks on girls' reputations. Gender joking in school classrooms and sexual harassment in higher education effectively keep most women in their place.

It is only since the early 1970s that male violence has come to be seen as a major social issue. Male control of sexuality according to some feminists is the foundation of men's power in society. Women face various forms of sexual harassment and violence in their day to day lives. Liz Kelly presents the idea of a continuum of violence between everyday sexual harassment and sexual abuse and shows how typical and aberrant behaviour shade into one another (Kelly 1988). She also points out that much behaviour women experience as abusive is not defined as a crime. Seventy-five per cent of the sixty women she interviewed did not feel safe on the streets, and 25 per cent of those who had access to a car felt the same. One-fifth never felt safe.

Girls in my research frequently mentioned the danger they feel on the streets and from boys:

> It's more dangerous for a girl than a boy to go out by themselves. A boy can go anywhere and just enjoy himself but a girl can't really, she's got to worry. Old men come along and molest you.
> Q *Has that ever happened to you?*
> Yes. I got followed home from school. It was only six o'clock. This man followed me down a dark alley. You always think someone is following you. The only thing is to kick them where it would really hurt and make them double up.

You can't trust a boy.

Parents are also very concerned about their daughters' safety. Michaela told me that her dad works with someone whose daughter had been gang-raped by her boyfriend and another of his friends at a club. The girl was distraught. He had stopped Michaela going to clubs as a result.

Violence in Adolescent Relationships

Little attention has been paid in the past to violence in dating relationships. More recently there have been a number of investigations into the dating experiences of adolescents (see Levy 1991; Roscoe and Kelsey 1986; Holland et al. 1991), and 'campus' rape is beginning to be acknowledged in American and British universities. It has been estimated that 50 per cent of rapes are perpetrated against adolescents, with the vast majority taking place between people who know or are dating each other (Levy 1991). One American study finds that 83 per cent of college women respondents reported having been victims of sexual aggression, 61 per cent since beginning college (Kanin and Parcell 1977).

In a recent British study (Holland et al. 1991) involving 150 young women in London and Manchester between the ages of sixteen and twenty, nearly a quarter of the sample reported having had unwanted sexual intercourse in response to pressure from men. These pressures varied from mild insistence to intercourse with threats, physical assault and child abuse.

The girls I interviewed talked about sex as something that 'happened to them'. The language of sexuality both silences women's expression of their desire and positions them as the object of desire. As Hannah says:

> You might be at a party and someone just dragged you upstairs ... And the next thing you know you don't know what's happening to you.

Girls frequently talk about being pressured into sex. Sometimes, as in the above example, there is no question that the sex was consensual, though the girls did not necessarily define it as rape. It is perhaps too simple to regard the boys as totally blameworthy. They are also locked into regarding girls in a contradictory way. On the one hand there are pressures on them to regard girls as conquests and to 'make' as many girls as they can; on the other hand they may genuinely like the girl. Yet their view of female sexuality is also affected by the images of the virgin and the whore, which lead them to treat women as objects and to regard their own sexual urges as out of their control and the woman's fault. This may be why the rape of even a virgin or a respectable married woman, as is described historically in *The Rape of Lucrece*, is still regarded, if not as the woman's fault, at least as a taint on her character. This is rooted in the power relation where if women are respectable (i.e. married or cohabiting) they require protection, but if not, then they deserve everything they get.

In a book on sex education in schools in Britain, Carol Lee described how when she asked classes to role play a court case where a fifteen-year-old girl has been raped, the boy was never found guilty by a class, whatever the circumstances. Assumptions were made that if the girl was coming home alone at eleven p.m. she must be a slut, or that if she was not a virgin then that meant that 'she really wanted it'. Whenever rape was discussed there were at least a couple of boys who said: 'But women really want it, Miss,' or, 'You have to knock them about a bit for them to enjoy it.' She described (Lee 1983) the following conversation with a fifteen-year-old boy:

If she didn't want [rape] she shouldn't have asked for it.
TEACHER *Why do you think she's asking for it?*
Well, look at the way she's dressed, showing tits and things.
(*They are looking at a picture of what would be called a liberated woman in a well known magazine. The woman is dressed respectably in a shirt – though without a bra – and baggy trousers.*)
TEACHER *You show your tits wherever you like – no one attacks you for it. Why should a woman be forced to wear a bra?*
She's doing it to get men.

TEACHER *But even if she were doing it to attract herself a boyfriend – and what's wrong with that? – does she deserve to be raped for it?*
If she's asking for it – Yes.

A girl is in a no-win situation: if she does not bother about the way she dresses she will be cast off as unattractive and un-feminine, but if she does look attractive she is in danger of being raped. This passage shows how rape, far from being the act of psychopathic sex-maniacs, is the extension of the normal oppressive structure of sexual relations.

It is a mistake to regard this as a problem of boys or men misreading the girls' signals. This type of analysis misses the power dimension endemic in sexual violence. The boys cannot fail to understand that the girls are 'saying no' and do not mean 'yes' unless they are totally clueless. More likely, they are unable to take no for an answer, because they refuse to recognize that she has the right to refuse. The condoning of violence implies that it is all right if the boys do ignore her refusal.

Youth Culture

Until fifteen years ago, the violent imagery and rampant sexism of boys in youth-culture studies were accepted with a degree of complacency that is quite shocking. Angela Mc-Robbie criticizes Paul Willis for failing to comment on the extreme cruelty of the boys' double standard and to show how images of sexual power are used to bolster boys' self-esteem. The misogyny is stark:

One teacher's authority is undermined by her being called a 'cunt', boredom in the classroom is alleviated by the mimed masturbating of a giant penis and by replacing the teacher's official language with a litany of sexual obscenities ... What Willis fails to confront, I think, is the violence and underpinning of such imagery evident in one lad's description of sexual intercourse as 'having a good maul on her'.

McRobbie draws attention to the closing lines of the book,

when Paul Willis gently probes Joey about his future, and he replies: 'I don't know, the only thing I'm interested in is fucking as many women as I can, if you really want to know' (McRobbie 1978:41). I have also mentioned the appalling way boys talk about menstruation and Julian Wood's picture of how some boys describe one of the boys' sisters.

Ten years on, in *Louts and Legends* (Walker 1988), the sexism among some young men in a study of Australian youth culture reflects a similar picture of the association between aggression and sex, but not all the boys agreed that violence was an appropriate way of treating a girl.

B Well, I'll tell ya, this girl named Y, right?
A My girlfriend.
B His ex-girlfriend. She dropped him.
WALKER *She's Greek?*
B Yeah, she's Greek . . . I'm gonna go over there tomorrow an' I'm gonna go [*pelvic thrusting*] . . .
C Fuckin' mole!
B That's what I'm gonna do; I swear it, I promise. And I'm gonna do that [*smacks hands together hard, indicating a slap*].
A See, listen. I don't know, he's got a different attitude to girls. I personally don't hit girls. It's against my religion, you'd say. So I don't like hitting girls. He, he – I don't know – somethin' different. He likes hitting girls. Like, if they do somethin' bad to him, he'll hit 'em, you know?
WALKER *Do you hit them a lot?*
B Well, I went to the beach one day, in the night. And uh, she took off her bra, right? I wanted to touch her boobs. She hit me here 'n' I went pow! pow! pow! [*C laughs loudly*] I hit 'er, she was on the ground and she goes, 'What did you hit me for?' Shut up mole [*slaps hands together*].

Walker in commenting on this argues that the violence is bound up both with anxiety about the sex/gender relation in masculinity and the desire to prove maturity as a man by contemptuous contrasts with others who decline to enter the macho contest. He fails to explain, however, why anxiety should necessarily lead to violence or why being mature and macho go together.

In one of my boys' groups, boys divided girls into girls who wanted sex (slags) and nice girls. But they clearly did not think that a girl should have sex unless she really wanted it: she should not just have sex to meet male sexual needs. In other words, they were not only against pressured sex, they did not want her to have sex just to please them. This is a very encouraging sign that at least some boys are respecting girls' subjectivity.

Yet you can see how boys are both affected by the objectification of girls, who they divide into 'slags' and girls who they like. Paradoxically, Sam would only have sex with a girl he did not like.

> BOY I It's not difficult to find a girlfriend, it's difficult to find a good one, one you can trust who's not interested in just one thing.
>
> Q *So what's a girlfriend you can trust like?*
>
> B1 One who's not there just for one thing. One you can talk to.
>
> B2 Or who maybe has good parents. 'Cos that rubs off [*laughter*] – no, honestly, it does.
>
> Q *So what did you mean one that's not just interested in one thing?*
>
> B1 Sex.
>
> Q *So there are girls who are just interested in sex?*
>
> B2 Put it this way, you can get girlfriends just for sex and you can get girlfriends who just wouldn't want to, but it's difficult to find one in between. Some girls you wouldn't want to have sex with 'cos you like them so much even if they wanted to, but you might know that they don't really want to, but they do it just 'cos they like you a lot. I can't explain. Do you know what I mean, Sam?
>
> SAM Yeah, someone who wants to please you, but they don't want to really.

Q *You wouldn't have sex if you really like the girl?*
SAM 'Cos I wouldn't, that's the way I am.
BI So you have certain girls that you like and there are ones who are sex objects.

There is a certain contradiction in the use of the word 'slag' in that it is used both to imply an object and a subject. A 'slag' is in sexual terms the woman who is fucked and discarded; however, it is also one of the few words to imply active female sexuality. The term is of course highly derogatory, yet it refers to a woman who behaves in the way men are expected to behave. A slag is a woman who is 'after one thing', someone 'who does not really care' or 'has sex for other motives' than love (the whore who has sex for money). This is relevant to the construction of female sexuality. The loss of virginity represents a cheapening of the woman, her value has fallen. Indeed in some cultures a loss of virginity would preclude the possibility of marriage. Secondly the implication as Paul Willis points out is that unleashing the woman's desire can lead to uncontrolled promiscuity. In analysing the term slag as a representation he comments: 'Woman as a sexual object is a commodity that becomes worthless with consumption and yet as a sexual being, once sexually experienced, becomes promiscuous.'

Willis, while allocating little enough space for an analysis of the term as used by his 'lads', does perhaps go the furthest in reading the term as a representation. But this reading falls short precisely because it fails to take up the significance of the term as the location of both worthlessness and sexuality. Locating the site of female sexuality in the slag is to both remove it from would-be non-slags and to ensure it is deemed bad, since the term represents 'a dirty person', unclean both literally and sexually and is akin to the term 'whore', thereby carrying all the connotations that surround it. By outlawing all active female sexuality, female desire is controlled and rendered unspeakable.

Willis recognizes the suppression of explicit sexuality in

women and attributes 'a half recognition' of this to the 'lads' who, he argues, fear that the opening of the floodgates of female desire will lead to promiscuity. Why is only one of the questions this raises about the construction of masculine desire around a sexual object that is attractive because it is untouched; discarded once consumed; then re-sought having become generally 'available' but denigrated?

The Effect of Unemployment

It is worth considering the extent to which the onset of long-term unemployment is likely to increase aggression and violence. According to Youthaid (1992), unemployment among the under-twenty-fives has risen by over a quarter of a million since July 1990 and is now at a rate of 16 per cent, compared to the national average of 9 per cent. Those unemployed aged under twenty-five, including sixteen- and seventeen-year-olds, total 864,000. In 1975 approximately 60 per cent of sixteen-year-olds were in employment. In 1992 the figure is around 10 per cent. Due to numerous government changes in the methods of calculation of unemployment rates, this figure must be regarded as an underestimate.

The socio-economic trends, referred to in the introduction, have led to a crisis in gender relations. Paul Willis (1984), in a series of articles written in the mid-1980s emphasizes how the socialization of young people into gender roles is tied to the transition from school to work and the acquisition, by males especially, of the wage. He speculates on the consequences of loss of work for the traditional sense of 'working-class masculinity'. He considers two possibilities. One is that traditional male working-class identity might actually be softened when the link with wage labour and the dignity and sacrifice of manual work is broken. Alternatively, the loss of the wage might lead young males to a 'gender crisis' to which one solution 'might be an aggressive assertion of masculinity and masculine style for its own sake'.

Anne Stafford (1991) undertook a participant observation study of unemployed girls and boys in government youth training programmes in Scotland in the late 1980s. She spent five months in a training workshop, two and a half months with boys and two and a half with girls. She encountered a completely different situation to that described ten years earlier by Willis (1977). The labour market had radically changed. Willis' boys were confident they could find manual jobs – his question was why they embraced them. For the young men Stafford interviewed even dead-end jobs were out of reach. She explained what effect this seemed to have had:

Boys' feeling of inadequacy, the sense of failure they felt about their lives, was also put on to a preoccupation with sex, 'scoring' and undermining girls. In a world where there were so many material hardships for these boys (bad housing, no jobs and no money), the way they lived and laughed through their difficulties was in many ways admirable. Yet it is difficult to hold on to and appreciate these positive things when so many of the ways in which they coped with their own situations were marred by sexism (Stafford 1991:59).

Her conclusion is disheartening. She found her young men appeared to be retreating into aggressive sexism, rather than moderating it: 'In all the times I was with the boys, I do not think I ever heard a girl discussed in terms of anything other than her appearance or as an object of sex. Girls as people were never mentioned . . . Girls were pieces of anatomy, to be discussed and commented on. Scoring and undermining girls were constant themes' (Stafford 1991:60).

The girls and boys inhabited different worlds, different spaces and did different jobs. Sex segregation reinforced the superiority of boys and subordination of girls. Stafford found that the whole culture both inside and outside the town was laced with sexism. From television, cinema, porn videos, and from their friends and relatives, they absorbed abusive and objectified images and messages about women. Stafford argued that as the material conditions of men's and boys' lives worsen, these tend to escalate and be exaggerated. She sums up her experience in the following way:

The overwhelming memory I took from the boys' workshop was of sexism. Their daily references to and treatment of girls as objects to be used and abused, their scathing disregard and contempt for anything feminine, tainted everything that happened there. Boys' culture seemed harsh and brutal in relation to girls. Success came in terms of alienated 'scoring' and objectified sex. Girls' culture in the area of personal relationships could not have been more different . . . Overwhelmingly they wanted boyfriends and long-term relationships (Stafford 1991:61).

We have seen how masculinity is inappropriately constituted with qualities of dominance, competition and superiority. Regrettably, until this changes it is likely that the economic recession will lead to an increase rather than a decrease in male violence. An aggressive masculinity combined with unemployment could well lead to an increase in the level of domestic violence faced by women. In a study of married couples Jan Pahl concludes: 'It seemed that there might be an association between the violence and the unemployment of the husband. Twenty-four per cent of the men were out of work when they committed the assault which forced their wives to go to the refuge: this was at a time when the unemployment rate in Britain was round 6 per cent' (Pahl 1984).

This conclusion as regards males is also borne out by a study of unemployed young people in the Isle of Sheppey:

For male youth the material and social bases of masculinity were undermined – they had no status as wage earners and no money as consumers. Consequently the symbolic expressions of masculinity were sometimes exaggerated. This was done in two main ways: through status-enhancing gestures or activities and through the retelling of such gestures or activities later as stories . . . These stories described such things as heroic and otherwise irrational acts of delinquency, great orgiastic binges of drinking or drug-taking, dramatic confrontations with the police, employers, the DHSS and others in authority. As well as recounting dramatic confrontations such stories also tended to glorify accounts of self-destruction and 'excessive' hedonism (Wallace 1985).

Weiss (1990) argues that in a deindustrialized America white working-class males are so threatened by their loss of traditional masculinity along with loss of job opportunities that the New Right is very attractive.

The consequences for girls are important. If young men, in response to long-term unemployment and the absence of the wage, are beginning to seek more symbolic gestures to confirm their masculinity, then young women, it seems likely, will face no let-up in the constraints on their own behaviour in the public sphere and social life which result from the activities of boys. Indeed an increased emphasis by males on the symbolic aspects of gender relations and masculinity could lead to an intensification of the types of constraints on women which we have looked at in this study. On the other hand it does seem that girls are beginning to question their secondary status and are becoming less willing to tolerate it.

Unemployment will have effects on girls too. Wallace argues that for a working-class girl lack of a job condemns her to the status of a junior within the home, and it is more likely that she will be given domestic chores to do as well. Tensions within the family as a result of unemployment may act as a pressure on girls to leave home and set up on their own. Often this may involve getting pregnant, getting married or both. Thus Wallace found that 'It was no coincidence, perhaps, that girls who had been unemployed for longer than three months out of their five years after leaving school were twice as likely to have left home, to live with a man, have children or get married than those who were regularly employed' (Wallace 1985).

Is Male Sexuality Uncontrollable?

Male sexuality and men generally are depicted as naturally dominant over women. Male and female sexuality are conceptualized in very different ways and the difference is falsely attributed to biology. Male sexuality is seen as a force of natural energy that seeks release, it is heterosexual and involves a progression from arousal to penetration and orgasmic release. It is a bit like a missile – once launched there is no stopping it, and the launching is the arousal phase. Harry O'Reilly, a retired New York police officer, comments wryly about this idea: 'How can a man argue that a woman "led him beyond his endurance"? Whoever heard of anyone dying of an erection? Men have been suppressing erections since time immemorial ... The idea of the "terminal erection" is a myth we have been perpetuating for years' (O'Reilly 1984).

The mistaken idea that male sexual urges are uncontrollable, that men are naturally promiscuous and are therefore not responsible for their sexual behaviour, and that aggression is a biological attribute of masculinity all contribute to the encouragement and exoneration of men from responsibility for their sexual behaviour. Several American studies (for example, Koss and Leonard 1984) indicate that men share in the belief that women are responsible for both stimulating and satisfying men's sexual urges.

Attitudes to Violent Behaviour

Various American studies have indicated that male violence is widely condoned. Miller (1988) reported that fifty-six of the adolescent girls he interviewed agreed that under certain circumstances it is all right for the man to use force to obtain sex. Miller and Marshall (1987) found one in every six women interviewed reported that they believed that when a man became sexually aroused it was impossible to stop him or for him to stop himself. Twenty-seven per cent of young women interviewed said they had had unwanted sex because of psychological pressure from boyfriends. They saw these experiences not as rape but as part of 'what happens on dates'. Sexual prowess and male violence serve as a means of symbolically proving manhood, which is seen as what men 'by nature' are. If men are sometimes a bit rough, overcome by their sexual urges, or provoked by women in some way, women have only themselves to blame for not taking avoidance action. Judge Pickles, a British judge, epitomized this view when in a TV interview he said, 'Every man has a bit of Jekyll and Hyde in them or a bit of the beast . . . When he is bad he's terrible – he's Jekyll and Hyde, all men are perhaps.' The distinction between 'rough wooing' and downright coercion is difficult to prove in trials and both in the USA and Britain only about 16 per cent of reported rapes result in a conviction (Steketee 1989, Wright 1984). Some women may still regard it as part of women's duty to satisfy a man's sexual urges.

Ways of Minimizing and Excusing Violence

Some girls are adamant that they will retaliate and not put up with violence within a relationship, but a common response to the predicament of a girl being beaten up by her boyfriend is for girls to see the solution to the violence in the girl's response. It is she who should avoid the violence or escape from it. Rarely does a girl condemn the boy's behaviour. Excuses are often put forward for why the boy should have behaved in such a way, some insinuating that the girl provoked the attack. On no occasion does a girl decry the prevalence of violence from boys. It is taken as 'one of those things' that is unchangeable. Not that girls should put up with it, though. Witness this discussion:

> SANDRA If someone hit me I'd turn round and strangle them.
>
> JANE And me.
>
> SANDRA I cannot understand people who stay with men who hit them.
>
> ZOE Some people do, though. Some girls say, 'Oh, he

hit me last night,' and I say, 'Did you hit him back?' And they say, 'No.' I say some people like being slapped.

HANNAH Some people do, though. Some girls say, 'Oh, he hit me last night,' and I say, 'Did you hit him back?' And they say, 'No.' Then I say, 'Are you still with him?' And they say, 'Oh yes.'

SANDRA I don't like that. I hate seeing boys hit girls.

HANNAH I wouldn't stick with anyone that hit me.

The difficulties a girl faces in breaking up with a boy are rarely acknowledged. Jean explains:

After a boy chucks you or you chuck him, you feel like life isn't worth living. You have no one to go out with. It's really depressing.

Dating violence is often referred to and usually condoned:

SANDRA [The boys] do it without realizing it.

JANE Sometimes someone really gets hysterical. They get annoyed and go, 'Shut up, shut up,' and 'That's it.'

SANDRA I think what probably happens with, like, husband and wife, they'll start an argument, and he doesn't mean to hit her really. He doesn't want to hurt her. It's just the last resort.

The danger of such violence is underestimated and excused by girls. When Jane objects to her boyfriend kissing another girl, and is hit by him, she still excuses his behaviour:

We just shouted at each other and he walked out after hitting me, but he had too much to drink anyway, but we got over it.

Other excuses for boys becoming violent are presented:

If a boy can't stick up for himself he comes to you just because you're a girl. He says, 'You've been telling my mates I can't stick up for myself,' and he hits you just to prove it to his friends. But he can only hit a girl 'cos he knows the girl wouldn't hit him back.

Girls often excuse boys for being violent on the grounds that they 'didn't mean it'. Even here, where Trudi thinks the boy is wrong, she cannot actually bring herself to attack him:

> It depends how he hits you. Like, if he's just messing about hitting you, or if he's serious. Like boys nowadays . . . Say, like, if he asks you out and you don't want to go out with him, he slaps you. I don't think that's right.

Rationales for violence appear without any condemnation of the boy's behaviour, and range from 'He doesn't mean it,' 'His friends are bullying him,' 'He needs someone to take his anger out on,' and 'He has had too much to drink,' to 'being provoked beyond endurance', or 'He does it because he loves her so much.' This mirrors Angela Browne's findings (1987) that male respondents who assault partners in serious premarital relationships often insist they were 'goaded' into the violence, claiming their assaults were the result of jealousy and perceived rejection. Women who have had no experience of violence in the past tend to view the incidents as isolated occurrences, attributing them to particular circumstances or stresses in daily life, rather than suspecting that this for their partner might be a characteristic way of relating. These women attempt to change their own behaviour. When this fails this kind of attribution leads to feelings of helplessness and depression.

Severe violence and rape are referred to by a number of girls:

> I've got two friends that have been raped and I've heard vivid details of their experience when they were raped and that really did terrify me. But then it sort of wears off. Before you know it you are walking around late at night asking for it. It's frightening. I do get worried about it, if it's late at night, if it's after a party. My boyfriend will take me straight to my doorstep. He would never leave me half-way home and head off home. He'd never do that.

There is a need to confront the many ways that men deny or fail to take responsibility for their violence. These include minimizing the violence, projecting blame on to the victims by claiming 'contributory negligence' (it's her fault), claiming loss of control, blaming alcohol or drugs, or citing internal or external stress as causes of violence. Men's attitudes and expectations toward their wives usually indicate an intent to devalue and denigrate rather than an intent to understand their wives. Rather than report what she actually said, the abusive man will characterize her words and actions in a mocking, trivializing or otherwise denigrating manner. Such rationales for male violence deny the woman's experience and are a way of condoning it. Girls are anxious to explain the boy's behaviour but not to criticize it. Another popular explanation is the cycle of violence:

> Like, if their mum got beaten up by their dad and they most probably end up taking it out on their wife or take it out on someone else and most probably end up taking it out on their wife or somebody like that (or if they are on their own with a prostitute) and take it out on her and beat her up just for the sake of it, just like that.

But girls know that violence is prevalent in many of the marriages around them and are anxious to avoid such a fate:

> There's one thing I don't like about what men do to their wives is beat them, at least that's what it's like with the next-door neighbour. She's not married and they're her children and her husband when he comes home at night sort of thing he beats her, just for the fun of it, and then he wants to go to bed with her afterwards. Like I asked her, you know, like, the other night she gets it just because he didn't come home the night before. There're silly people like that and that's why I don't want to get married.

Girls generally regard a girl as responsible if she allows the boy to behave in a chauvinistic manner – gravely underestimating the relatively powerless position she is in. By treating the man and woman as equal in the relationship, her subordinate position is denied. Debbie, aged sixteen, who lives with her mother after her parents divorced, is confident that she can avoid domination:

> I think like in a relationship with a man it's really up to

you and if you're going to let the man you're with walk over you, do what he likes, go out with his mates and you have to sit at home, well, on the whole it's your fault 'cos you're a person and you can get up and say, 'No, I want to go out, I want to do this, I want to do that.' When it comes to jobs, it is unfair, the pay and other things, but when it's like a man and woman relationship – it's both people who have got to try. Like I know people who'll say they've rung up Tony or whoever and he says, 'Oh, I'm going out with me mates,' and they'll say, 'Oh well,' and they won't go out. I think that's wrong. Why should you sit at home waiting for someone when they've gone out having a good time? Either you should say, 'Oh, I think that's really very nice' – or in looking for a boyfriend you want someone who's not going to go off with his mates and expect you to sit at home.

Here Debbie recognizes the unfairness in the job market, where men attract higher wages, but somehow imagines that at home equality reigns and the man and woman are on equal footing; that as long as they both try all will be well. She does not question why it is that the man has a place to go, the pub, to meet his friends, whereas girls have few places, money to spend or cultural support for going out. She does not question that if she has children, it is she who will be expected to look after them when he is out at the pub, and it will not be acceptable for her to go out on her own. In spite of this, Debbie blames the girl who stays at home while her boyfriend goes out with his mates, but her only resolution is to look for a boyfriend who is not going to go off with his mates and expect her to stay at home. What she fails to mention is the constraints on girls having a good social life without boys – the few places they have to go without being molested, difficulties getting back late at night, greater control over them by concerned parents. All in all she fails to mention that it is men who dominate and control the public world where women are always at risk of harassment and are targets for verbal abuse. The irony is that Debbie blames the girl, not the oppressive state of sexual relations. If a girl is blatantly sexually harassed and denigrated, this is often written off as unpleasant but just 'boys having a bit of fun'.

The only recourse the girl who is dating has is to break off the relationship, which opens her up to the 'slag' categorization, as we have seen. Violence is largely condoned by the community and rarely seen as a product of very unfair relationships between the sexes.

Boys' violence can almost be turned into a positive quality, whereas 'violent' girls are described in sexually pejorative terms: 'bitch' or 'madam' (see Adams and Walkerdine 1986: 36). Certainly some boys in group discussions were blatantly open about sexual violence. Take this comment as to how to 'shut up girls':

> If you don't shut up, I'll slap my big dick in your face.
> Girls deserve to be hit.

Fighting is a common topic of conversation among boys:

> DAVE We have a lot of arguments.
> JUAN No nuclear weapons to back us up.
> DAVE We like starting trouble.
> JUAN Say you're on the street and another geezer pulls a knife out. You have to do something to him.

A group of Bengali boys complain that fights are part of day-to-day life:

> ZEBHIA If I wanted to play football with somebody, I'd have to fight for it.

When asked what fights were about, Zebhia replies:

> That you're big, man, I'm big, I'm tough, and I can fight. To show they can fight and they're strong and not to be messed with.

Research into Moral Judgements

Women have historically been regarded as inadequate morally, as incomplete in their moral development, at worst as dangerously irrational creatures who, if not controlled, are capable of disrupting culture and progress. Relegated to the private world of the family, women have been deemed incapable of abstract thought or the ability to make judgements on the basis of independent autonomous universal principles. They have been seen as irrational, unpredictable creatures whose biological body functions render them unreliable when menstruating. Women are not to be trusted because they lie and cheat to protect their husbands and children, regardless of the implications this may have for the wider social order. For this reason women have been seen as unsuitable for the priesthood, for the judiciary and for positions of authority. They are dependent and in need of protection because they are a bit childish and helpless. Women are seen as incapable of the detachment necessary for the highest forms of abstract moral discourse.

The tendency for girls to see violence as an interpersonal problem which the girl has to deal with, rather than condemning violence in the abstract reflects the way that girls have been shown to approach moral problems. It is relevant therefore to see girls' condoning of violence within this context.

Research into the development of moral behaviour indicates that there are differences between girls' and boys' moral judgements. Piaget (1965), who carried out extensive research into the development of cognitive abilities in young children, describes two stages of moral thinking, the stage of moral realism, where young children make judgements on the basis of the results of an action, and the stage of reciprocity, where the child makes judgements on the basis of the person's intention. For example, if a boy breaks two cups helping his mother with the washing up, this is viewed at the stage of realism as worse than if he breaks one cup on purpose.

Kohlberg (1981) elaborates this into six different stages of moral reasoning. His theory of moral development was developed from his studies of eighty-four boys whose progress he followed over twenty years. When measured on the scales he devised, women appear to be deficient, stuck at his third stage of development where morality is conceived in interpersonal terms and goodness is equated with helping and pleasing others. Kohlberg regards his fifth and sixth stages, where relationships are subordinated to universal principles of justice, as superior. He gave students hypothetical situations containing moral dilemmas and found that the essence of morality is different for girls and boys. Girls, he discovered, gave views about moral dilemmas in terms of interpersonal relationships or how the individuals involved would be affected. Boys on the other hand more often gave opinions which were made on the basis of abstract principles.

Carol Gilligan strongly refutes Kohlberg's theory that girls are less capable of principled moral reasoning than boys, or stuck at an earlier stage of development. She argues that Kohlberg's concept of stages is fundamentally flawed and that if one begins with women's lives and develops constructs from their experience, moral problems arise from conflicting responsibilities rather than rights; this requires a different mode of thinking, one that is contextual and narrative rather than formal and abstract (see Gilligan 1982:19). She differentiates between a 'self' that is defined through separation and a 'self' delineated through connection.

She gave teenage girls and boys Kohlberg's moral dilemmas and by analysing their replies came to a different conclusion. She argues that what Kohlberg had seen as women's moral weakness, manifest in an apparent diffusion and confusion of judgement, is inseparable from women's moral strength, i.e. an overriding concern with relationships and responsibilities. Girls show a reluctance to judge on the basis of universal principles of justice, which is indicative of the care and concern for others that infused the psychology of women's development. For example, Gilligan asked young girls and boys to give their view on the dilemma of how to reconcile responsibility to others with responsibility to self. Jake, aged eleven, argued that 'you should go about one-fourth to the others and three-fourths to oneself'. He then went on to argue that 'If what you want is to blow yourself up with an atom bomb you should maybe do it with a hand-grenade because you are thinking about your neighbours.'

Gilligan points out that the imagery of violence, depicting a world of dangerous confrontation and explosive connection as opposed to a world of care and protection, a life lived for others whom 'you love as much or even more than you love yourself' was striking. To Jake responsibility means not doing what he wants because he is thinking of others. To Amy, the eleven-year-old girl Gilligan interviewed, responsibility means doing what others are counting on her to do regardless of what she wants. Girls therefore see morality as a way of solving conflicts where no one is hurt. For boys fairness and autonomy predominate.

Exactly the same process can be seen in the way the girls view violence in their relationships. Not one girl put forward an argument that violence was wrong in principle or that boys should be punished for being violent. The way the moral problem is viewed is in terms of how male violence should be dealt with within the context of relationships. The danger here is that violence is accepted as an inevitable part of life or something that girls cannot do very much about except to try to avoid it if they can. Unfortunately many of the strategies of avoidance involve forms of subordination of which girls appear to be relatively unaware. I would take issue with Gilligan that such modes of thought are therefore necessarily a strength. It is important that women contest their condoning of male violence, so damaging to their interpersonal lives.

Bullying and Suicide

In May 1992 Kathleen Bamber, a sixteen-year-old British schoolgirl, hanged herself. She had been taunted at school and had told her mother that she was being made fun of and called names. She had kept a diary describing how she had been bullied. Kathleen's parents, together with the television presenter Esther Rantzen, started a national campaign against bullying. Esther Rantzen commented, 'Having read the suicide note and part of her diary, I know she was driven to despair by the bullying she experienced, and killed herself because she found it painful and humiliating.' The chair of the local education authority denied the pain the child had suffered and schools have done little to counteract it.

Schools need to include in the curriculum the facts about bullying. They need to develop assertiveness training. They need to ensure that more care and skill go into the design of school buildings and playgrounds. Children should be encouraged to speak out. In 1992 more than a thousand boarding-school pupils rang a telephone help-line complaining of bullying and sexual abuse, often by teachers.

According to recent reports there is a growing realization that much bullying is verbal and can lead to tragedy. Verbal taunts often play a key part in an adolescent's decision to commit suicide. Anna explains the process:

> In the first year everybody starts off dead quiet but as they grow up they start. They stroll around and see who they can pick on, anything that comes to mind. Even if what you wear is not to their liking they talk about you and everybody starts joining in, just to be big. Often they're jealous.
>
> Q *What are they jealous of?*
>
> I don't know really, they just want a lot of attention. They start spreading rumours. Like, this girl I had an argument with, she went around saying that I was calling these other girls names and they just start trouble.

Anorexia and bulimia can be seen as ways of attempting to gain control of impulses that are denigrated by a peer group and society. Or a girl may turn her anger inwards and take drugs or even contemplate suicide.

The difficulty men have in expressing their feelings, particularly feelings of worthlessness, in a society where the model of masculinity they are presented with is no longer adaptive, may account to some extent for the dramatic rise in suicides among young men. Figures from the British Youth Council report (1992) show that the most common causes of death among young people under twenty-five are linked to accidents and violence accounting for 61 per cent of deaths of males and 37 per cent of females in the 15–34 age range in 1989. This is double the 1951 rate. The fastest growing suicide rate according to the Samaritans' latest figures is among the under twenty-fives – up by 41 per cent in the last decade. Of all young suicides, four-fifths are male, but of all those attempted four-fifths are female: one girl in a hundred aged fifteen to nineteen attempts suicide every year. One in five of the gay teenagers interviewed in Trenchard's and Warren's research (1984) had attempted suicide. Every four minutes a young person aged under twenty-five calls the Samaritans. In the last thirty years the number of suicides by young people under the age of twenty-five has trebled from 214 in 1958 to 629 in 1988. It is likely that the actual rate of suicide is higher, as coroners may bring a verdict of accidental death to save the parents from the stigma of a suicidal death. The rising suicide rate among young men is likely to be connected to the rise in youth unemployment. This is an area which needs more research.

Policies on Sexual Harassment

Visiting a comprehensive recently the first thing I heard on entering the gates was a girl discussing boys with her friends: 'All they do is call us slags.' Little seems to have changed over the past five years and schools, as Halson found, appear to sanction rather than challenge sexual harassment. 'Whilst smoking, wearing denim clothes and boys wearing earrings are regarded as inappropriate behaviour for students at Henry

James School, calling girls slags, for example, is not' (Halson 1989:139).

Sexual harassment and violence are areas that badly need to be addressed. Carrie Herbert (1992) produced a handbook on sexual harassment for teachers, students and parents where she points out that although the national curriculum does not specifically mention harassment, there is a clear commitment to equal opportunities and scope for this to be included in Education for Citizenship (National Curriculum Council 1990). She outlines how to write and implement a policy regarding sexual harassment, various curriculum initiatives and personal strategies.

Schools have policies on violence, but this rarely includes sexual violence, and when such incidents come to teachers' attention they are trivialized or dismissed. Myra, one of the girls I interviewed, described how she was blamed for sexual abuse about her being plastered on the toilet wall. When I asked her what was written she replied:

That I was a slag and so on. Then on Monday there it was again. The PE teacher got people scrubbing the toilet walls. Later I was looking for my little sister after school and the PE teacher says to me, 'Myra, come here.' I walked over to her and everyone's standing there thinking, 'What's she want with her?' And she says to me, 'I've just had people cleaning the walls and isn't it funny how your name comes up so many times.' She says, 'You know what toilet I'm talking about?' I say, 'Yeah.' She says, 'Do you know who done it?' And I can't really tell her who done it, especially with everyone looking on, so I say 'No.' So she says, 'If I see your name written up there again you and your friends are gonna get into trouble.' So I said, 'Well, it was nothing to do with me.' She says, 'Well, if that was my name written up there I'd have it scrubbed off.' So I said, 'It's in great big green felt pen.' She goes, 'Let me see your name up there again and there'll be trouble.' She thinks I'm going to walk all round every toilet in the breaks scrubbing everything off the walls. I tell my dad. He said to tell her in future to find the idiots who wrote it and make *them* scrub it off. It really did annoy me.

The teacher, by focusing on Myra, is blaming her for having her name on the wall. Teachers are not encouraged to use such opportunities to challenge the use of verbal sexual abuse and denigration of girls. Instead Myra, a victim rather than a perpetrator of the abuse, is blamed and reprimanded for the incident.

Why do teachers rarely intervene by challenging the terms of the abuse? Valerie Walkerdine (1990) in her study of primary-school teachers describes how female teachers downplay and ignore the reported violence of boys – violence that is frequently directed at them as well as the girls. This downplaying – indeed, downright approval – of boys' violence is endemic to the pedagogic and child-rearing practices on which it is based. That is, boys are independent, brilliant, proper thinkers. They are also naughty. There seems here to be a splitting: the teachers downplay the violence of boys, transforming it into words like 'naughty', understood as a positive attribute on the basis of independent thinking. On the other hand girls are, by and large, described as lacking the qualities boys possess. They are no trouble, but then their lack of naughtiness is also a lack of spark, fire, brilliance (Walkerdine 1990:127).

In this way Walkerdine argues that violence is not simply condoned but linked to a certain kind of mastery. This gender difference according to Elshtain (1983) is associated with the social organization of gender into the public–private split that has created two polar types: the 'beautiful soul' and the 'just warrior'. The beautiful soul resides in the private sphere and represents all that is pure and beautiful, and the warrior defends the beautiful soul from violence. Ruddick (1983) links this with two types of cognitive styles, the abstract and the concrete. The concrete concentrates on the personal and detailed and the abstract is depersonalized and oriented around generalization. The latter style makes it possible to create an abstract enemy, for example the 'Gooks' as the Vietcong were named by American servicemen during the Vietnam War, and kill them without moral anxieties. This is far more difficult to accomplish in the concrete style, because the enemy is seen in terms of its human qualities.

Gender Joking Initiated by Men

School staff rooms too are sites of 'gender joking' and denigration of women teachers. Cunnison (1989) observed staff of mixed sexes in a senior comprehensive school over a three-month period. She observed great hostility to feminists. She analysed the role played by gender joking in maintaining the comparative success of men and the failure of women to gain promotion within the school management hierarchies. Several studies (see Delamont 1980, Ball 1987:67, 79) indicate that gender is a major correlate of school position. Jokes focus on femininity, woman's domestic role and sexuality. Some refer to women's appearance and thus to conventional ideas about gender and femininity. For example, when a woman raising funds for the PTA asked people to estimate the time she would take to run a mile, one man she approached responded that he would rather estimate the size of her bust (Acker 1989:153).

Some jokes are put downs, where women are defined at work in sexual, domestic or maternal terms. This can be seen as a way of subordinating and controlling women. A major source of the power of these jokes is that they refer to cultural stereotypes or ideal images of women that are largely shared by both sexes. Women do care what they look like; they do want to be sexually attractive and do want or have children. Cunnison suggests that various tactics are used to resist women's promotion and to designate competency as an indication of lack of femininity. Women were caught in a double bind. She describes how one young teacher with excellent prospects was referred to jokingly as an SOB (son of a bitch).

A woman teacher criticized her temperament as cold, that is, in conventional terms unfeminine, and suggested that her future as a woman high up in the male hierarchy would be lonely and isolated. There is also a commonly held view that women do not have the same right to promotion, as they can always return home to their husbands and be supported by them.

Three responses to this 'joking' can be differentiated, though all ran the risk of indicating that 'women are unable to take a joke'. Such remarks were greeted by silence, though sometimes with facial expressions ranging from resignation through exasperation to scorn. Secondly, some women played along with the 'joke', which required a quick wit and the ability not to take offence. Lastly the stereotypes were occasionally challenged by, for example, ridiculing the male chauvinist. One feminist teacher attached stickers – 'YB a wife' and 'Is there life after marriage' – to the backs of selected members of the staff room. Caroline Ramazanoglu (1987) outlined 'the routine insults, leers, sneers, jokes, patronage, bullying, vocal violence and sexual harassment' that academic men use to keep 'uppity' women in their place and the difficulty in getting such behaviour recognized as harassment.

Pro-feminist Programmes Regarding Violence

Violence among boys is often condoned, yet sex-education classes rarely address the issue. Feminist approaches that have been developed in the USA challenge men's violence and the traditional therapeutic interpretations that see the problem of male violence as a family problem. EMERGE, which was set up in 1977 in Boston, involves a coordinated community approach involving services for women, men's programmes and coordination of criminal justice and social-service agencies. Pro-feminist programmes directly challenge men's violence. A fundamental principle is to make men responsible for their violence. The appropriate use of confrontation is crucial. Confrontation involves attempts to persuade men to acknowledge their violent behaviour and to accept responsibility for actions and for the need to change (see Dobash and Dobash 1992:244). These are the kinds of programmes which need to be introduced into schools both in the USA and in Britain.

In this chapter I have illustrated how sexism is not only rampant among young male adolescents but is endemic in school staff rooms and in society at large. The sexist objectification of women and girls, noted by sociologists such as Julian Wood and Paul Willis in the 1970s, does not appear to have abated or to have been modified. Anne Stafford's research indicates that everything the adolescent boys she observed said is suffused with sexism. Though not all the boys in my project are blatantly sexist, fighting and the double standard are part of the largely taken-for-granted context of most of their lives, of their friendships and of their masculine status. A few boys are in favour of greater equality, but they are in danger of being labelled 'wimps' and 'poofs'.

In the last ten years economic changes, the world recession and the resultant restructuring of the economy are enforcing marked changes on young people's lives. Unemployment among youth is increasing and the mark of masculinity, the breadwinner role, is no longer available to many young men. It is however too simple to conclude that unemployment or economic conditions in themselves are the cause of increased violence. Though violence may appear to be more prevalent in certain sections of the community, and it may appear to be class related, this is not necessarily the case. Male violence against women and child sexual abuse occur across all classes. Violence also takes different forms in different social groups. The covert violence of politicians who advocate war and domination rather than negotiation and conciliation emanates from the same constitution of masculinity as domination and control.

It appears that in this crucial period of adolescence when identities are being formed violence in the form of pressured sex and verbal sexual abuse is condoned by many, though not by any means by all, boys, but it appears to be largely uncontested by teachers and is rationalized as 'the way boys are' by many girls, and even celebrated in popular films, videos and pornography. The results of this could be disastrous. As the recession deepens, and young men are increasingly thrown into unemployment, they may fall back on other ways of asserting their masculinity. Some young men are genuinely confused as to what is expected of them, yet the new man is more myth than reality. As the economic façade of ever-increasing economic growth fades, the inappropriateness of the macho model of masculinity will become more apparent.

The condoning of male violence and domination has even wider moral implications relevant to the way that our educational and political systems are constituted and operate. The same sexist vocabulary of sexual 'conquest', objectification and domination, the prioritizing of abstract principles such as 'fighting for democracy', can lead to a legitimation of war and militarism regardless of the human consequences. It is not by accident that we speak of the rape of the countryside as well as sexual rape.

In the next chapter I will outline the forms of resistance that young women are adopting in opposition to their subordinate status.

Bibliography

Acker, S. (ed.), 1989, *Teachers, Gender and Careers*, Fulmer Press

Adams, C., and Walkerdine, V., 1986, *Investigating Gender in the Primary School: Activity-Based Inset Materials for Primary Teachers*, Inner London Education Authority

Ball, S., 1987, *The Micro-Politics of the School*, Methuen

Blumenthal, M. D., et al., 1972, *Justifying Violence: Attitudes of American Men*, University of Michigan, Ann Arbor

British Youth Council, 1992, *The Time of Your Life? The Truth about Being Young in 1990s Britain*

Browne, A., 1987, *When Battered Women Kill*, Free Press

Cunnison, S., 1989, 'Gender Joking in the Classroom', in Acker, S. (ed.), *Teachers, Gender and Careers*, Fulmer Press

Delamont, S., 1980, *Sex Roles and the School*, Methuen

Dobash, R. E., and Dobash, R. P., 1992, *Women, Violence and Social Change*, Routledge and Kegan Paul

Elshtain, J. B., 1983, 'Beautiful Souls and Just Warriors: Reflections on Men, Women, War and Cultural Image', paper presented at the Thematic Panel on Gender and Politics at the Annual Meeting of the American Sociological Association, Detroit

Gilligan, C., 1982, *In a Different Voice*, Harvard University Press

Halson, J., 1989, 'The Sexual Harassment of Young Women', in Holy, L. (ed.), *Girls and Sexuality: Teaching and Learning*, Oxford University Press

Herbert, C., 1992, *Sexual Harassment in Schools: A Guide for Teachers*, David Fulton Publications

Holland, J., et al., 1992, *Pressured Pleasure: Women and the Negotiation of Sexual Boundaries*, Tufnell Press

Kanin, E. J., and Parcell, S. R., 1977, 'Sexual Aggression: A Second Look at the Offended Female', in *Archives of Sexual Behaviour*, 6, pp. 67–76

Kelly, L., 1988, *Surviving Sexual Violence*, Polity

Kohlberg, L., 1981, *The Philosophy of Moral Development*, Harper & Row

Koss, M., and Leonard, K., 1984, 'Sexually Aggressive Men', in Malamuth, N., and Donnerstein, E. (eds.), *Pornograpahy and Sexual Aggression*, Academic Press

Lee, C., 1983, *The Ostrich Position*, Writers and Readers Lesbian and Gay Youth

Lees, S., 1989a, 'Blaming the Victim', *New Statesman*, 24 November 1989

Lees, S., 1989b, 'Trial by Rape', *New Statesman*, 1 December 1989

Levy, B., 1991, *Dating Violence: Young Women in Danger*, Seal Press

McRobbie, A., 1978, 'Working-Class Girls and the Culture of Femininity', in *Women Take Issue*, CCCS, Women's Studies Group, pp. 96–108

Mahony, P., 1985, *Schools for the Boys*, Hutchinson

Miller, B., 1988, 'Date Rape: Time for a New Look at Prevention', in *Journal of College Student Development*, 29, pp. 553–5

Miller B., and Marshall, J., 1987, 'Coercive Sex on the University Campus', in *Journal of College Student Personnel*, 28 (1), pp. 38–47

National Curriculum Council, 1990, *Curriculum Guidance 3: The Whole Curriculum*, York

O'Reilly, H., 1984, 'Crisis Intervention with Victims of Forcible Rape: A Police Perspective', in Hopkins, J. (ed.), *Perspectives on Rape and Sexual Assault*, Harper and Row

Pahl, J., 1984, *Private Violence and Public Policy*, Routledge and Kegan Paul

Piaget, J., 1965, *The Moral Judgement of the Child*, Free Press

Ramazanoglu, C., 1987, 'Sex and Violence in Academic Life, or, You Can Keep a Good Woman Down', in Hanmer, J., and Maynard, M.(eds.), *Women, Violence and Social Control*, Macmillan

Roscoe, B., and Kelsey, T., 1986, 'Dating Violence among High School Students', in *Psychology*, 23 (1) pp. 53–9

Ruddick, S., 1989, *Maternal Thinking: Towards a Politics of Peace*, Beacon Press

Stafford, A., 1991, *Trying Work*, Edinburgh University Press

Steketee, G., and Austin, A., 1989, 'Rape Victims and the Justice System', *Social Services Review*, University of Chicago Press, Vol. 63, No. 2

Trenchard, L., and Warren, H., 1984, *Something to Tell You*, London Gay Teenage Group

Walker, J. C., 1988, *Louts and Legends: Male Youth Culture in an Inner-City School*, Allen and Unwin

Walkerdine, V., 1990, *Schoolgirl Fictions*, Verso

Wallace, C., 1985, 'Masculinity, Femininity and Unemployment', unpublished paper presented at the Sociology of Education Conference, 1985

Weiss, L., 1990, *Working Class Without Work: High School Students in a Deindustrialized Economy*, Routledge, Chapman and Hall

Willis, P., 1977, *Learning to Labour*, Saxon House

Willis, P., 1984, in *New Society* 29 March, 5 April, 12 April 1984

Wright, R., 1984, 'A Note on Attrition in Rape Cases', in *British Journal of Criminology*, Vol. 254, No. 4, Oct.

Youthaid, 1992, in *The Time of Your Life?*, British Youth Council

Chapter 7
Strategies of Resistance

Perhaps the most positive effect of changing our linguistic practice will be to destroy the pernicious belief that we have to be controlled and oppressed by our language. Once over that hurdle, we can start learning to speak out with confidence and to use the resources of language and metalanguage, so often denied us or used against us, in the continuing struggle against patriarchy.

(D. Cameron 1985:173)

To speak as an act of resistance is quite different than ordinary talk, or the personal confession that has no relation to coming into political awareness, to developing critical consciousness.

(bell hooks 1989)

Girls have to develop a feminine identity in line with their cultural ascription, but to become a person in their own right they need to develop an identity in contradiction to this. From the onset of menstruation, girls have to deal with the contradictory messages about their feminine identity. Girls' identities are fractured by the widespread depiction of them as sex objects, yet indications of sexual desire on their part can render them as 'whores', 'good-time girls', and 'slags'. Adolescent socialization for girls is fraught with discontinuity and conflict. Girls are supposed to be interested in boys, yet many boys still expect them to behave in traditionally female ways. Girls are aware that such feminine behaviour renders them subordinate both in the private and public worlds and some girls are rebelling against such subordination.

This chapter examines the greater restrictions placed on girls at adolescence and the different strategies girls adopt to deal with the double standard. Girls are not passive victims but are daily constructing complex strategies for contesting the language and abuse that render them subordinate. As I suggested in the introduction, gender is not simply reproduced: girls' reactions to these processes of subordination are complex and contradictory. Their resistance is limited by the language available to them. Calling a boy a slag, for example, which some girls said they did in retaliation to boys' harassment, carries no bite. Individuals are rendered powerful or powerless depending on what language they have access to. Finally, their insubordination also activates a backlash, as it threatens not only male power but also the masculine identity to which it is constituted in opposition.

I illustrate the way girls deal with contradictory messages that reflect the pressures on girls at a time of great social change. The fundamental contradictions are between career and marriage and children, between autonomy and self-sacrifice, between sexual attractiveness and promiscuity, between sexuality and motherhood. Girls have to pave a way through these contradictions and strive to form an identity in a society that is still beset by double standards of sexual morality which pervade every area of a girl's life – relations with boys, friendships, schoolwork, the public world and social life.

As we have seen, at school girls are encouraged to work hard and plan a career, yet developing academic interests carries the risk of rendering them unfeminine and unattractive to boys. They are expected to be independent, and yet working-class girls still have to undertake domestic and caring tasks to a far greater extent than their brothers. They are expected to have boyfriends, but it is they who are held responsible for using birth-control, even more crucial in the nineties with the risk of AIDS, and their reputations are under constant surveillance. As we have seen in the last chapter they even hold themselves responsible for male violence. Some girls end up feeling confused and ambivalent, lacking in confidence and self-esteem or out of control, as indicated by the rising figures of anorexia nervosa. But change is underway and many girls are contesting the taken-for-granted sexism around them.

Most girls fluctuate in the extent to which they embrace the attributes of femininity, and some girls are redefining femininity more positively to involve less submissiveness. Acquiescence to femininity can be seen as leading to submissiveness, passivity and low self-esteem. Rejection of femininity can involve being written off as too tight or a lesbian. A few girls in more progressive schools are able to come out as lesbians. In order to avoid the stigma still strong in most schools, most girls pave a middle way, exhibiting both daily resistance and daily accommodation (see Walker 1983). Girls' responses to their objectification fluctuate and are often contradictory. Girls do not always passively accept being called names; they often challenge boys. Sometimes they resist using practices of refutation, refusal and subversion but sometimes the weight of common sense becomes too great and they decide it is easier to ignore it or try to prove the boy is wrong about them. But abuse sticks and often worries girls and reduces their self-esteem. It is through these practices that the social structure is created and recreated. For many years girls were brought up to develop 'only' a woman/female identity directed to the reproductive function and caring for a husband, with a subjectivity that was constructed as muted or suppressed. Self-sacrifice was the hallmark of womanhood. Today such clear delineation has gone and what comprises womanhood is misty, confused and contradictory.

Girls may adopt different practices at different times. At one moment girls accept sexual abuse as natural and fail to contest its terms, at another they contest the terms of abuse that macho boys adhere to. Though girls are not always aware of the processes that render them subordinate, they are aware of the pitfalls and problems of relating or not relating to boys, and they spend inordinate amounts of time and energy concerned with this dilemma. How to navigate one's way through the system of gender domination is a major problem for girls. The overall effect of sexual abuse on girls shakes their confidence in themselves and can lead to depression, eating disorders and other disturbances.

Greater Restrictions on Girls

Many girls resent the restrictions (sometimes called 'protection') placed on them from entering the public sphere and the pressures to conform to the feminine role. Most girls soon become aware that their position is different from their brothers'. Parents place greater restrictions on girls as they approach puberty and often do not explain why their activities are being monitored. Linda describes how boys' lives are different:

> They get away with more. They've got less responsibility. It's not the same, it's not the same for a girl. Like my brother gets away with much more than what I would when I was his age.
>
> Q *What kinds of things?*
>
> Getting in – what times – when I was his age I wasn't allowed to walk in at all times like he walks in. I don't know, it's like, boys themselves. It's everyone around treats them differently to girls. And they say 'I'm a boy!'

At school, all the girls agree that boys can get away with much more than girls. Outside the home restrictions are placed on where they go and how late they can stay out at night. bel hooks, an American feminist, describes how she used to go as a child with her father down the street with its barber shops, pool halls, liquor stalls and pawn shops, and that when she approached adolescence her mother put a stop to these trips. She describes how by her teenage years she had learned to fear this world.

I no longer felt the intimate sweet companionship with strange black males and even the old familiar faces. They were the enemies of one's virginity. They had the power to transform woman's reality – to turn her from a good woman into a bad woman, to make her a whore, a slut. Even 'good' women suffered, were somehow always at the mercy of men, who could judge us unfit, unworthy of love, kindness, tenderness, who could, if they chose to do so, destroy us (hooks 1989:149).

A girl is taught that her appearance is crucial to her identity.

She learns that her body, if controlled and disciplined, is a passport to success. Girls must be slim, must restrict their body movements and behave demurely, sit with their legs firmly together rather than spread out, and avoid eye contact with any man they meet in the street. They are taught that they should not take up much space nor talk too much. In other words they are taught that the public sphere is not their territory and they can enter it alone only at their own risk. You simply have to glance in the average pub, restaurant or sports stadium to realize that men control the public arena: it is men who dominate the public sphere. At a time when boys are encouraged to play sport and develop their bodies to their full potentiality, girls are taught that their bodies are something to be ashamed of, that suffer emissions of blood that they must at any cost conceal and that they cannot be free to roam the streets or to go around without fear. Finally, girls gradually become aware that men view them in a contradictory way, either professing desire and passion for them, or at the other extreme denigrating them, putting them down and treating them without respect. Girls' responses to this demarcation are not uniform and most girls respond in different ways at different times.

Several women writers have outlined the pressures they experienced when adolescent. Nawal el-Saadawi, an Egyptian feminist, in *Memoirs of a Woman Doctor* movingly outlines how she resisted the path that had been ordained for her in adolescence. How she resented having to grow her hair longer and longer, and have it twisted into plaits and imprisoned in ribbons while her brother, with his hair cut short, could run and play. She resented always having to ask if she could go out, unlike her brother who was given a free rein and she cried her eyes out because she knew she was a girl who was being socialized into dependence. She resented that 'everything in me was shameful' and blamed God for favouring boys in everything. She resented developing breasts once she realized that that was where men's eyes rested, and that was what a dirty old man in the park, who grabbed at her one day when she was sitting innocently on a bench, wanted. How she rebelled, she cut off her hair, refused to get married, left home and became a doctor (el-Saadawi 1988). Simone de Beauvoir likewise felt the same indignation about her subordinate status. She saw no rational reason why, if men should sow wild oats, women should not be subject to the same rules. At seventeen she believed that both parties in a relationship should have an equal vote in how the relationship should develop (de Beauvoir 1963:190)

Strategies

Girls adopt strategies all the time; not only when they are actively assaulted but in their day-to-day interactions with boys. Insufficient attention has been paid to the way young women react to harassment or to the effect this has on their developing subjectivity. I have separated the strategies girls adopt to deal with everyday sexist abuse, both physical and verbal, into three categories. Conformity involves broadly accepting the terms of abuse, failing to question the double standard and joining boys in calling other girls 'slags'. It involves conforming to the status quo. When verbally abused this strategy will lead a girl to try to 'prove' that the abuse is not true, to deny it. Avoidance involves changing behaviour to avoid abuse, either physical or verbal, or ignoring the verbal abuse. Lastly, tactics of resistance, involving verbally subverting or challenging the terms of the abuse on the one hand and collectively resisting it on the other, will be outlined.

Conformity

Some strategies, though understandable, lead girls to collude in their own subordination. Conforming strategies often have the effect of leading girls and women to blame themselves rather than to contest the abuse, as we saw in the chapter on violence. How girls respond to abuse is crucial to the meaning it embraces. The reason why calling a boy a slag is ineffective is because it is not relevant to the boy's reputation. But girls can turn the tables on the boy by subverting the double standard. Unfortunately most girls are so concerned about their reputations and the double standard is so much part of common sense that their most common response is to deny that the label applies to them, accepting therefore the validity of attacking a girl's reputation.

Denial can take a number of different forms. It can involve denying that boys are different in any way and trying to fit in with them. Tracy describes how she treats girls and boys as similar:

If I like a girl then I treat her, you know, like friends, and if I like a boy, the same. There's no difference for me. Perhaps I mean if you really like a boy or something you'll treat him a bit different, but you're not gonna be sort of unnatural.

Bridget, a middle-class girl, has no feelings of inferiority:

I'm for women's lib. I think I'm just as capable, far more capable than a lot of boys. I know I'll get a good job and it annoys me when they start presuming that just because you are a girl you're not as good as them.

Even these girls, who see themselves as equal to boys and are incensed about the double standard, are often rendered powerless when faced with verbal abuse. Rather than contesting boys' use of such words as slag or dog, the most common response of girls is to try to find evidence to prove that they do not fit into the derogatory category. So Kate says:

I've been walking down the street and someone's said to me, across the road, being rude, and says, 'You slag,' and I think, 'How do you know? You've got no evidence.' That makes me angry, 'cos, like, you see someone and you're meant to know whether they sleep around or not.

Here Kate is angry that the boy calls her a slag without having any evidence. Even when the boy does not know her, a girl reacts by denying the accusation rather than by objecting to the use of the category. For them what is important is to prove that you are not a slag: what they unquestionably accept is the legitimacy of the category of slag. In other words, the category has an uncontested status. Compare this with when Stephen describes his reaction to being called a poof:

I'd tell them to shut up basically.

When asked whether he would say 'No, I'm not,' he says:

I might say, 'Prove it.' But generally we just have a laugh and run each other down. We'd be more likely to use less offensive words.

Q *Like what?*

For instance, something like, 'Your house is so dirty the mice moved out,' or something like that, I've heard being used . . . Or you might say, 'You've never had a girl-friend.'

Other boys would not be called on to refute the accusation and generally the boy would shrug the insult off. Girls, on the other hand, never seem to be able to do this. So Wendy, asked what she would do if someone called her a slag, replies:

I'd turn round and say, 'Why? Tell me why?' And then if they said, 'Because you were with so and so last week,' then if I'd liked them I'd just say, 'You knew I liked them. I was just unlucky enough for them to chuck me. It's not my fault. It just happened. It's not as though I did it just for sex, just because I wanted someone to sleep with that night.'

Here Wendy argues that she would need to explain herself and prove that she had not slept with the boy just for sex but because she had liked him and that it just 'happened'. Her use of the word 'happened' is interesting, as it implies that she was not really responsible. What she fails to take up is the iniquity of the boy's accusation. The implication is that what makes a girl a slag is having sex with a boy 'just for sex', without really caring about the boy, which is of course exactly what the boys are encouraged to boast about, and what makes them 'men'.

For girls to have such sex in this way makes them prostitutes. Another analogy between the construction of sex with
prostitutes and 'voracious' male sexuality is that both involve
separating their bodies from their emotions. The problem
becomes one of proving your 'innocence', when proof is always
contestable, never clear-cut.

Even when accusations do not specifically relate to actual
sexual behaviour, proving one's innocence often involves
referring to other girls to find out whether the accusations are
valid or not. This is where girls are drawn into policing each
other. The discussion of power does not relate to whether girls
and boys are concentrated in certain roles rather than others,
but can be seen as a field of force in which girls are equally
trapped rather than something exercised by boys over girls.
Girls exercise power over other girls by ostracizing those they
consider to be slags and by constantly monitoring each other's
reputations. If a girl denies the accusation, whether or not she
is believed will depend therefore on the strength of her relationships with other girls. But even then her friends will want to
find out whether the accusation is true. The real difficulty is
proving to other girls and boys that the accusations are false.
Michelle explains what a girl in this situation can do:

> She could have a go at him, show him up when he's with
> everyone, confront him with it when he's with his mates,
> and make him feel little.

She then goes on to discuss what happens when this occurs:

> Danny – this boy went out with one girl and then met
> another girl straight afterwards and he was meant to
> have said he had had both of them, and they both went
> at him together and really had a go at him. She told us
> she was shouting at him saying, 'Oh, you've had me then
> have you? Funny, I never knew about it,' and saying
> things like that. But even then it could have been true
> and they could have been lying. They could show him
> up. But he could say, 'Well I did. I did y'know.' He
> can't prove it and he can't disprove it, can he? But say

she had slept with him, right, to get herself out of it she could just go up to him and say, 'Oh, so you've been spreading it around that you've slept with me,' in front of his mates, 'but you haven't.' He can stand there saying, 'But I have, I have,' and they'd never know who to believe, would they?

It seems the boy is more likely to be believed. What is important is producing the evidence. As Sharon points out:

... A slag is usually someone you know and you just have evidence of what they've done.

The result of having to maintain a good reputation, means that girls have got to be very careful with whom they socialize. This applies not only to girls at school. In Holland and Eisenhart's study of women at two American universities, one with a predominantly white and the other a predominantly black intake, it is suggested that

It is not so much what one actually does with a man but how whatever was done might be presented detrimentally by other women, if they found out about it. The special way in which romantic relationships made women vulnerable to loss of respect, especially among other women, led them to be especially vigilant to control what other people knew about their romantic relationships (Holland and Eisenhart 1990:116).

In closely knit American campus environments, women put much energy into maintaining respect and controlling information about personal relationships and emotional investments. This appears to be a major factor in female friendships being weak and secondary to relationships with men. Black women students are more emphatic about the need to be reticent about their emotional affairs and the difficulty of being able to trust other women. Once they have found a boyfriend, they only spend time with girlfriends when their boyfriends are not available. As we saw in the chapter on friendship, girls often drop their girlfriends when they get serious with a boy.

Resignation

Girls sometimes react to being blatantly sexually harassed with resignation. Grossly sexist behaviour is seen as merely stupid rather than insulting and threatening. The boy may not be criticized for his behaviour: his chauvinism is regarded as natural and unalterable. In a similar vein, his infidelity is viewed differently, as Jessie recounts:

> JESSIE It doesn't seem so bad for a boy. It seems natural for a boy when you think about it [*laughs*]. You just think it's normal but for a girl it ain't.
>
> Q *You don't think it's normal for a girl?*
>
> JESSIE No, I think in the end girls end up to be prostitutes and I think that's wrong.

Jessie's laugh when she says that it is natural for a boy to be unfaithful suggests that she is aware of the contradiction, but she immediately rejects the idea that girls and boys should be held equally responsible by slipping back into the conclusion that this would lead the girl to prostitution, which is 'wrong'. The boy's behaviour is morally immune: it is natural. Where does her reasoning come from and how can she let the boy off the hook in this way? The taken-for-granted insolence of boys is evident in many accounts:

> Like, this boy was calling me a bitch. I don't know what he was calling me a bitch for. He was picking on me. 'You bitch,' he goes. He knew my name. He just wanted to make fun or something 'cos he had some friends round there. He comes up to me and he says, 'Hallo, sexy.' I goes, 'Who are you talking to?' 'You' . . . I was scared and 'cos my friends were there we just walked off. So stupid, fancy calling someone a sexy bitch.

The most common form of conformity is to get a steady boyfriend. All the girls agree that if someone starts to get a reputation, the one way they could avoid it is to 'get a steady boyfriend': 'Then that way you seem more respectable like you're married or something.' A boy is often seen as lending protection to a girl:

> Say you have a boy protecting you. It's as if no one can hurt you or nothing. You're protected and everything. If someone does something to you, then there's him there and it just makes you feel secure.
>
> Q *What do you need protecting from?*
>
> He doesn't like it when other people are out to get you. It doesn't mean that other people can't do nothing to you but it's kind of protective toward you.

The need for protection emerges in a number of interviews. Charlotte, in describing how her brother is treated differently from her, attributes this to his ability to protect himself because he is a boy:

> Boys are a totally different physique. I could go out and I could be raped whereas he couldn't. He'd have more chance of protecting himself. I think that comes up the whole time. It's not that a boy is more trusted. It's that he's freer.

Being on your own holds fears for many girls – some related to the harsh reality of existing in a male-dominated world where protection is needed. Girls can never go out on their own or even with girlfriends without the ever-present fear of assault:

> I don't like going out. You feel safer if you go out with other girls than go out on your own. You're even safer with a boy, that's what you feel whether it's true or not.

Avoidance

All girls learn about avoidance from early in adolescence, as bel hooks so vividly describe above. Avoidance can involve restricting one's movements, not going where you want, avoiding certain streets, markets, whole areas of the town, less public areas of the park, the pubs and even the street. Avoidance means not sitting on the top of buses unless they are crowded, avoiding sitting next to a strange man, avoiding empty carriages on trains and keeping an eye on who gets on and off so you do not find yourself alone with a man, avoiding the glances of men, avoiding going into a pub on your own, and crossing the road if you think you are being followed. It involves constant surveillance. Certain boys and men are dangerous, although you can never be certain who to avoid. Avoidance involves not going out after dark, not coming home on your own after a party, not taking a taxi or minicab on your own. It involves curtailing independent behaviour, not going to the movies, a disco, being careful what you drink. As Jenny explains:

> It makes you feel terrible, makes you feel as if you don't wanna go out, say, soon as you go outside the door you get someone calling you a slag. It's not worth it.

At its extreme avoidance can take the form of agoraphobia, which can be seen as a projection of women's feelings of loss of control, a parody of the social restrictions placed on them. In projection the individual fails to recognize herself as the agent of the feelings, but attributes the fears to an outside source, such as threats in the outside world.

In one of the most popular novels of the 1970s, *The Women's Room*, Mira, the main character, realizes that the dice are loaded against a woman going out on her own. She is dating Larry, but after a row over whether or not they should have sex, which she does not feel ready for, he abandons her in a bar. She dances with his friends, has too much to drink and narrowly escapes being gang-raped. It is then that she realizes that she can never be free:

She could not go out alone at night. She could not in a moment of loneliness go out to have a drink in company, she could not even appear to be lacking an escort, if that escort decided to abandon her she was helpless. She couldn't defend herself. She had to depend on a male for that ... She averted her eyes from any male who passed her and never smiled at them even when they greeted her ... Her dream of choosing and living a life of her own had vanished (French 1978).

Some girls do go out on their own regardless, but the fear of being sexually harassed places real constraints on a girl's freedom.

Girls often prescribe ignoring insults:

> Most boys are bullies. They say, 'Oh, look at that slag,' and just call you names. It's best not to lose your temper and take no notice of them, 'cos silly people like that are not worth taking notice of.

A few girls decide to avoid boys altogether. Haylee and Maggie explain:

> If a boy does ask us out we say, 'No, don't want to know,' because we want a career and go round the world and all that. We just leave them alone . . . We talk to some boys and they always go around with girls, so if [the girls] see us they start calling us names and it will aggravate us and we would not be able to get on with our work, so we just tell [the boys] to go away.

> I don't really bother with boys now − just get on with my homework. I go out with my friend and then go back home. I was brought up not to like boys really, 'cos I've heard so much about what they do − robberies, rapes and all that, so I keep away from them.

> Q *What do you mean − brought up not to like them?*

> Well, my mum told me never to go with them because they damage your health and things like that, don't know what she means, but she says they ruin your life if you get pregnant. She said it's best to keep away from them, so I do.

The danger of avoidance is that you can then get the reputation for being a lesbian or too tight. More explicitly, boys talk of being 'tight-legged', in comparison to slags who 'have their legs wide open'. The girl can't win. If she avoids boys rumours may spread that she's really tight and boys will whisper, 'Oh God, she's really tight. It's pointless going out with her. She's no good.'

Girls also talk about the need to avoid boys if a girl begins to get a reputation. Better still, getting engaged is a greater protection. Avoidance can also involve avoiding girls who have a reputation. Girls fear contamination:

> If someone for whatever reason has got a bad name, either your dad doesn't approve or she's got a bad name or whatever you can't go with that girl.

> Because you get called the same name; if you're hanging around with a slag you must be one.

Resistance

How possible is it for girls to resist the categorizations and labelling, and escape from their force? The responses of girls to verbal abuse mirror the three kinds of resistance that Tajfel (1978) put forward in a theory of social identity, which he argued developed from ingroup-outgroup relations. He suggests three kinds of activity can be adopted by subordinate groups to challenge the power and authority of dominant groups. Firstly, social creativity, which is where the subordinate group seeks to create a new or positive image for itself. Arguments that womanliness is superior to manliness or that the idea of woman embraces a degree of autonomy combined with feminine qualities of caring are examples of this activity within feminism. Girls in my research do not seem to be able to think clearly enough about traditional femininity and are too confused about the contradictions in their lives to adopt this position. What is more relevant are Tajfel's two other reactions. Assimilation or merger is where the subordinate groups adopt positive features of the high-status groups they wish to join. This as we shall see is the tactic adopted by the tomboys. Lastly, social competition is where subordinate groups seek to change the relative power and status of groups by active or passive resistance.

The questioning of taken-for-granted practices of everyday life is an essential first step to bringing about change. The potency of calling a girl a slag rests on the anxiety girls experience about their sexual reputation. Ignoring insults can be an effective way of counteracting the abuse. If girls can recognize the double standard, then they will not be so shaken by it. Yet being independent in thought or deed carries risks. Being free and independent can signal promiscuity. The freedom of women can be equated with prostitution. What is lacking is a language through which the legitimacy of slag as a way of censoring girls can be contested. As Anna describes:

> Boys can sleep around and aren't called anything, but girls who do are called slags.
> Q *What do you think about that?*
> I think it's unfair discrimination – but that's the way it goes.

On the other hand if a girl goes out with one boy and sleeps with him 'she will be called a nice girl' (boys talking). Or, as Madeleine says:

> If a girl sleeps with two different people then she's considered a slag, but if a boy does it's good. I think it's really bad. It really annoys me. I call boys tarts.

Girls talk about calling boys 'tarts' in retaliation, but applied to boys such insults have no cultural meaning, so the word makes no impact. Sexist abuse is effective as girls feel vulnerable about their reputations. It is not just that a girl loses respect from boys, but also from girls, who may ostracize her and spread rumours about her too. This militates against any form of collective resistance.

Another way of gaining acceptance is to behave in a way that is sexually neutral in order to be accepted in a masculine activity. An example of this is given by Anne Stafford in her study of a youth-employment scheme in Edinburgh. She describes how Trish, who was trying to be accepted into an entirely male paint workshop, learned fast when it came to what was and what was not acceptable behaviour. To be allowed to stay she had to be seen as sexually neutral. She created a role for herself that was helpful to everyone. The moment she relaxed, however, and her relationship with the boys eased, she began to see them as potential boyfriends. She immediately became a sex-object and was seen as available, causing the workshop to buzz with excitement. When she flirted, the boys' behaviour went unsanctioned, but hers was judged on a different standard and her reputation was badly affected (see Stafford 1991).

In some senses education treats girls as if they were boys. Valerie Walkerdine points out how a clever girl is treated as though she might be male (possessing a phallus), while she has to negotiate other practices in which her femininity is what is validated (Walkerdine 1990:46).

Julia is aware that 'it is up to you'. Some girls are successfully redefining femininity to include a degree of activity. It is possible to contest the essentialism so taken for granted. She describes the kind of girl she prefers:

> I like someone who is mostly active, doesn't like staying in or being bored all the time and wants to go out and enjoy themselves, and someone who is interested in being active, likes to play tennis, doesn't want to stay with their mums all the time.

Boys object to attempts to put boys down:

> I don't like a girl who runs you down for no reason. They're flash. They say, 'I like your jumper.' Whisper. Whisper. Girls who do a lot of talking behind your back.

Sexist abuse is so taken for granted that unlike racist abuse, which is now usually recognized as such, sexist abuse is still seen as normal and common sense. The power relations underlying such abuse are rarely recognized and any tendency to rebel is seen by men – and other women too – as unwarranted behaviour. Suzanne describes behaviour that she regards as showing off:

> One of these girls was walking down the road near our school. Somebody whistled to her, a man, and she turned round and waved. If that had been me, I would've just looked down and pretended it didn't happen. Even if there was nobody around I don't think you should turn around and wave, would you? It makes you think badly

of them, don't it? You think what kind of a home have they been brought up in? If I'd done that my dad would've given me a wallop I would never forget. I wouldn't do it anyway.

Q *What do you think it means?*

Giving him the 'come on' sign.

It does not occur to Suzanne that responding by demurely looking down renders the girl passive in the face of provocation. But any active response, even to such provocation, can render the girl a slag. Liz Kelly (1988) argues that if women challenge men and refuse to be controlled they risk a violent response from the men and are accused of provocation. Girls also risk being ostracized by other girls for being provocative. Here again it is the girls who are implicated in policing each other.

Girls must be passive and demure and walk with their eyes down. The chauvinism of boys on the other hand, though noticed, goes uncontested and is accepted as 'what boys are like'. As Cheryll says:

As soon as he's got [sex] from you he's off, just saying 'had my piece from her'. Off he goes and news travels around. Some boys like to boast about it.

Girls do seem indignant about 'boys mouthing' but yet many do not question it or think they have the means to resist the double standard.

Another form of resistance is to report the abuse to a teacher. Some male teachers are quite often openly sexist, even putting their arms round girls and making comments such as, 'You're looking gorgeous today.' Girls in Carol Jones's (1985) research talked of being sexually assaulted by male teachers:

I didn't really want to go to see Mr — but he said, 'Put your chair here, love,' and he kept reaching over me. I didn't know what to do.

Another girl reported, 'Mr — stopped me in the corridor and asked me if I had a school book, then tried to get me in the stock room. He said I was well developed' (Weiner 1985:29). Other teachers appear to find it difficult to challenge actively or question boys' sexism. By violating received versions of femininity, to provoke shock or embarrassment, girls face the opposition of other girls and possibly teachers.

Another tactic is for girls to try and create positive images of femininity by using their feminine charms, by exaggerating stereotyped femininity in order to create new positive images of femininity. The punk image of the 1970s is an example here, and Madonna also plays around with images of the slag: 'In our society a woman who is overtly sexual is considered a venomous bitch. So what I like to do is to take the traditional, overtly sexual bimbo image and turn it around and say I can dress this way and behave this way but I'm in charge. I call the shots. I know what I'm doing' (Madonna, TV Interview, 1991).

Humour is a common method of dealing with the abuse and several girls attempt to 'laugh off' incidents:

> Sometimes I go in the toilets and I see my name written up – 'Ann's a slag,' or something like that. I just laugh like if someone comes up to my face and told me I was a slag or a slut I'd just laugh. So long as you're not one, then you've got nothing to worry about.

Yet laughing off such incidents is no joke. Pat Mahony (1985) pinpoints the delicate line between regarding sexism as a joke and being pushed into reacting in anger. The common adage that 'women have no sense of humour' perhaps is rooted in this delicate balance:

At the time, I never regarded sexual harassment as a really major problem. It was more like a game which had developed from the infant and junior school with 'kiss-chase' and boys pulling up your skirt ... I only really began to get annoyed when it became more than a joke and started to happen all the time. I suppose the embarrassment annoyed me more than the act itself. If you're seen with boys continually chasing you, etc., then you get a reputation for 'liking it' (Mahony 1985:50).

Putting boys down is a more successful tactic. When I was interviewed on *The Jimmy Young Show* I was asked how girls respond to sexual abuse, as my interviewer said he 'had never met a girl who did not give as good as she got and could not stick up for herself'. The implication here is that any girl worth her salt can cope with the double standard. To do so on any other terms than to deny the accusation is to come up against the whole weight of taken-for-granted sexual morality. Girls talk about 'showing boys up in front of their friends', and, 'making them feel little'.

Fighting

Girls can react to taunts in the way that boys do by fighting. Anne Campbell, in her study of fifteen- and sixteen-year-old delinquent girls from working-class areas of London, Liverpool, Oxford and two areas of Glasgow, found that although they were the girls who are often the ones typically ostracized as slags, sluttish or common, they rejected the labels and condemned the idea of sexual easiness contained in them. She analysed what situations sparked off fighting and found that fights invariably arise from slurs on each other's reputation, such as 'slag', 'tart' and 'scrubber' (Campbell 1981). Eighty-nine per cent had participated in at least one fight. Questions about who had made the last remark before the fight revealed that the most commonly offered reason was that slurs had been put on their sexual reputation and insinuations made about their sexual morality.

She concludes that although girls' fighting is strikingly similar to boys', girls do not fight in groups to defend either their reputation or their territory, nor do they 'seek public arenas in which to demonstrate their bravery'. What she does not appreciate is that an attack on a girl's reputation is an attack on her personal morality and integrity, which only she can defend. She is often isolated in her defence. She cannot demonstrate that she is respectable by a display of bravery – only by convincing her attackers that she has not slept around. The trouble is that there is no way you can provide evidence. As Sally explains:

> You can't tell a slag from seeing someone walk down the road. I mean, you might see a girl walking down the street looking really debauched, sort of a mess, make-up's run everywhere, but you don't know the reason. You might call her a slag, but I mean she could have just been beaten up by her boyfriend – you don't know the reason. You should have evidence before you call someone a slag.

By no means all the girls approve of fights, and some regard them as childish. Rebecca comments:

> I hate to see girls fighting. It looks stupid. Girls like to scratch more and try to get each other's hair out, they don't punch.

While bullying and fighting by boys are recognized phenomena, investigation of the extent of girls' involvement in such activities has yet to be seriously undertaken. What is clear however is that girls' involvement in fighting is very much associated with conflicts over sexual reputation. Any attempt to deal with it therefore will not get far if it fails to tackle the root cause of violence – the domination of male concepts of sexuality and the ways in which these concepts lead girls into relations of competition and antagonism. Fights between girls are therefore less fights over boys or boy-friends in any direct sense than fights over personal reputation and integrity. It is this that makes them ambiguous and difficult to resolve. Fifty-five per cent of Anne Campbell's sample had no idea who had won in fights between girls. A reputation cannot be clearly and unambiguously redeemed even by physical victory in the same way as it can either by a boy proving his bravery or, for that matter, a clear competition between girls for boyfriends. But, ultimately, the very vacuity and ambiguity of the term slag is, as I have argued, a reflection of its role in the control, by males, of girls' freedom.

Sometimes, of course, competitiveness does play a part. In the following incident, boys were drawn into a dispute between two girls which led to one boy being thrown out of a top window and ending up in hospital. This supports Cheryll's view that fighting often arises when a girl has a grudge against another for fancying her boyfriend or being too popular. I came across several examples of girls drawing others into disputes. The most dramatic example was recounted by several girls: the fight had resulted in one boy being thrown through a plate-glass window and two older school-leavers being sent to gaol for assault. This is how Gita explains it:

> Jacky used to go to my primary and she got expelled last week. She had this big fight. She was one of them and everyone knew she was one, you know. One of that kind . . . Someone had written some bad language about her. She thought it was this boy Johnnie in our class. He fancied another girl, Rosie. So she beat Rosie up. She lost the fight because someone held her back. So she then called her brother around and everyone beat up Johnnie and threw him out of the window. Right out of the window, you know, through the glass. You know the double doors, one of them, they threw him through the glass.

When Gita was asked if fights were usually about that sort of thing, she replied:

> Usually about names, calling people bad names and, um, if they don't like them, usually this starts a fight.

Collective Resistance

Girls also find it difficult to fight the categorization of their friends:

> Q *Suppose you were in a pub and a boy started talking about one of your friends and calling her a slag. How would you react?*
> TRACY If we know for a fact that they're telling the truth, then we'll agree but if not, we'll stick up for them.
> JANE Well, not necessarily, 'cos the boys know if they've

done it or not, wouldn't they? You just say, well, it's up to her, and then find out from someone else. But if it was, like, someone said it about someone I knew wasn't like that, I'd stick up for her because I'd know she's not like that, so I'd say: 'No, you're out of order.'

Q *But if she was like that, but was a really good friend, you'd stick up for her?*

JANE No.

TRACY It's up to them if that's what they want. I don't agree with it, but it's up to her. It's her life. If she runs it that way not the way I want her to run it, that's up to her. Everyone thinks I'm a prude anyway.

Occasionally girls mention collective ways of dealing with sexual harassment which are successful, like this incident in the changing rooms:

The boys love coming into the girls' changing rooms when they're changing. This boy, right, we made a decision next time he comes in, grab hold of him and start taking his clothes off and see how he feels. All the girls were watching him. He never came back.

The failure or lack of opportunities for women to resist collectively, the opposition most likely to be successful in counteracting women's subordination, is rarely adopted. Ros Coward asks when feminism has identified and analysed discrimination: 'We are led to the uncomfortable question about women's own collusion in these oppressive structures, whether women have stood to gain anything from these structures and whether individual or class interests haven't simply overridden more collective concerns . . . Women have to face up to their own role in their oppression and not to accept easy answers' (Coward 1992).

This view underestimates both the lack of discursive practices of resistance for girls and the strength of the backlash when girls or women do resist their subordination. While it is true that girls rarely appear to attack sexism or question the morality of the boys' behaviour, this is due to the predominant view that it is natural for a boy to behave in a downright egotistically dishonest, bolshie, untrustworthy, unfeeling way. Girls are plugged into defending their reputation with all the odds against them. What characterizes the way 'slag' functions as a term of moral censure is that on the one hand it has uncontested status as a category, and on the other hand it has an elusiveness and a denigratory force. When girls do complain about the sexism of boys this opens them up to further attack.

Girls make distinctions between boys, and suspect there are not many boys who can be trusted. Behaving in an unfeminine way can also be pathologized, though some girls, as shown in Leah's case, manage to resist this categorization:

> I've been to the doctor about my temper, my bad attitude toward my parents and school, the teachers. He wanted me to see a psychiatrist but I wouldn't go. I just said, 'I ain't going. It's no good. Look, I said, I ain't mad.' I did, I told him. I said I ain't going.
>
> Q *What I don't understand is why you call it a bad attitude.*
>
> Well. I really get a bit cocky, my mouth. My mum says I got a big mouth 'cos I shout.
>
> Q *That's not unusual.*
>
> Yeah but I'm a bit flash as well.
>
> Q *What does flash mean?*
>
> Shouting and roaring around and that. Being bossy. Saying, she can go there and he can do that.

Institutions such as medicine and the law are involved in keeping girls to the accepted construction of femininity. Feminist criminologists have shown how the law discriminates against young women charged with status offences, that is, offences that depend on the juvenile status of the transgressor (see Datesman and Scarpitti 1977). Here the determination of a girl's 'incorrigibility' or 'uncontrollability' depends largely on the court's opinion. It has been consistently shown that girls are far more likely than boys to be charged with these offences and then to receive a harsher sentence for such behaviour, in spite of the fact that girls commit less serious offences, less often, than boys. It often appears that such charges are a way of controlling sexually active young women. The Director of the US National Centre of Juvenile Justice, Hunter Hurst, declared that:

The issue is that status offences are offences against our values. Girls are seemingly over-represented as status offenders because we have a strong heritage of being protective towards females in this country. It offends our sensibility and our values to have a fourteen-year-old girl engage in sexually promiscuous activity. It's not the way we like to think about females in this country. As long as it offends our values, be sure that the police, the church or vigilante groups or somebody is going to do something about it. For me, I would rather that something occur in the court where the rights of the parties can be protected.

Subversion

Feminists have been aware that the language of abuse can be subverted or eliminated. Radical feminists particularly have argued that language is man made (Daly 1978, Spender 1980) and have attempted to develop a 'feminist' language or way of 'subverting discourse'. Subverting racist language can also be seen as an effective form of resistance. bel hooks (1989) speaks movingly of the need to understand the power of voice as a gesture of rebellion and resistance whereby the oppressed are enabled to break their silence and speak out. Three examples of this in British schools spring to mind. Grace Evans (1992), a black teacher in a London school, described how West Indian pupils used patois as a means of subverting the school curriculum in response to the racism of teachers who disparagingly referred to them as those 'loud black girls'. In another study, groups of Asian girls resisted teachers' stereotypes that Asian pupils had language difficulties by insisting on speaking Urdu in class (Brah and Minhas 1985). Finally, in Mirza's study of African Caribbean girls in the late 1980s, black girls rejected and challenged teachers' low expectations of them (Mirza 1992).

Language has been seen as fundamental to women's oppression (see for example Irigaray 1985, Sellars 1991). Deborah Cameron convincingly refutes the argument that language is inherently male, but argues that the problem is not one of language but of power, which consists to a large extent in decoding what stories will be told. Women's talk is not inherently subversive but becomes so when women 'begin to privilege it over their interactions with men' (as in consciousness-raising groups). Men trivialize the talk of women not because they are afraid of such talk but in order to degrade it. Therefore women's talk will be harmless as long as women consider it trivial compared to talk with men. (Cameron 1985: 157–8). This argument links with Ardener's (1975) concept of women as a 'muted' group, in which he argues the dominant groups in society generate and control the dominant models of expression. Muted groups, he argues, are silenced by the structures of dominance. If they wish to express themselves they are forced to do so through the dominant models of expression, the dominant ideologies.

Any group that is silenced or rendered inarticulate in this way may be considered a 'muted' group, and women are only one such case (travellers, children, deviants are some others). Mutedness is the product of relations of dominance that exist between dominant and subordinate groups in society. Ardener's theory does not imply that the mutes should be silent, nor does it imply that they are neglected at the level of empirical research. Women may speak a great deal, their activities and responsibilities may be minutely observed by the ethnographer, but they remain muted because their model of reality, their view of the world, cannot be realized or expressed using the terms of the dominant male model. The dominant male structures of society inhibit the free expression of alternative models, and subdominant groups are forced to structure their understanding of the world through the model of the dominant group. The free expression of the female perspective is blocked at the level of ordinary direct language. Women cannot use the male-dominated structures of language to say what they want to say, to give an account of their view of the world. Their utterances are oblique, muffled, muted.

Ardener therefore suggests that women and men have different world views or models of society. We can see this occurring in the way a girl's voicing of sexual expression is disallowed. Even non-sexist men find it almost impossible to take on the dominant hegemony, as we saw in the chapter on sex education. It is through women's writing that change will occur. Cixous (1975), a French feminist, argues that women's writing will create an 'elsewhere' in which 'the other will no longer be condemned to death' and in which 'that something else (what history forbids, what reality excludes or doesn't admit)' can emerge.

There is, however, a sense in which if women take on the word 'slag' as subject rather than as object, it is possible to subvert the misogyny embedded in the term. Mae West and Madonna are stars who have subverted the term by applying it to themselves. Madonna's video company is named Slutco. She is a triumphant slut who challenges the derogatory meaning of the word and turns it into a symbol of female freedom. Nor is she unaware of the power involved in resisting male dominance: 'It's a great thing to be powerful. I've been striving for it all my life,' she asserts. Mae West too rose above the term and took on a dominant active role in her sexual relationships.

Madonna successfully subverts the meaning of 'slag'. She enjoys her sexuality and avoids being portrayed as a sex object. 'I'm not ashamed,' she asserts. Her body has radically changed shape and now resembles an athlete's. In an interview she told how her grandmother used to beg her not to go with men, to be a good girl. She plays on the madonna/whore dichotomy and declares that being sexual, being a 'whore', is fine. In videos she often plays two roles, one questioning the other as if debating the two views of female sexuality: the moral virgin versus the voluptuous slag. She sings voluptuously, dressed like a prostitute, making a mockery of her grandmother's and the church's view that women are either virgins or whores. In an interview she explains: 'If you can create yourself, you can recreate yourself.' Change is important because it means you have grown. By wearing a suit and monocle, she ironically subverts the constraints of being constructed as male or female. She dresses like a prostitute. She is successful at gently exploding myths. Take her contribution to the condom campaign:

> You never really get to know a guy until
> You ask him to wear a RUBBER
> Hi you, don't be silly, put a rubber on your willy
> (said on her 'Blond Ambition' world tour)

The use of the word 'willy' cuts the embarrassment and male obsession down to size.

Madonna has been criticized for exerting power only along traditional supremacist, capitalistic and patriarchal lines (bel hooks 1981). In the documentary *In Bed with Madonna* she reveals that she made the cast very dependent on her and treated a woman who came to her for help with considerable disdain. She chose a cast of characters from marginalized groups – non-white folks, heterosexual and gay, and gay white folks, and then publicly described them as 'emotional cripples'. bel hooks sums up by saying: 'All that is transgressive and potentially empowering to feminist women and men about Madonna's work may be undermined by all that it contains that is reactionary and in no way unconventional or new.'

Subverting masculinity carries this risk. Are women who successfully subvert the dominance wanting to be dominant themselves?

There are several examples of girls attempting to subvert the constraints of femininity by taking the initiative. Eileen describes one such episode when her friend Rita approached a boy she fancied:

> He has hair that comes down and flips back, it's light ginger, nicely shaded. He has dark eyebrows [*laughter*], I'll tell you what she did to him. I can never forgive her for this. We were walking along one dinnertime. Every dinnertime he had a pint of milk. She goes to him and says, 'Ain't you going to give Eileen a drop?' He turns round and puts the milk bottle down against the wall and she goes, 'You can't leave it there you know.' It right showed me up. I suppose that is what friends are for. At the time I did not find it funny but now I think about it it was funny. I just thought it was horrible. I thought she treated him wicked.

Rita in this episode is perhaps not really being subversive. Rita is being 'pushy' not on her own behalf, but on behalf of her friend. Thus this practice could be seen not as subverting but as ultimately consolidating the very practices they are contesting. There are few examples of girls successfully subverting or contesting the boys. Lilly describes how she tried to contest the way boys behaved as though they owned a girl by buying her drinks. Yet she does not think she managed to do this successfully:

> Some boys think they're flash because they've got a bit of money and think they can buy you. I said to one boy, 'Ditch your money,' and he wouldn't let me so I thought, 'He thinks he can just do what he wants.'

Then there are the tomboys, who are tough and cool and stand up for themselves and consider themselves as good as boys. Some girls adopt the stance of boys bragging to take the mickey out of a group of conventional girls. This group is failing to resist the boys and trying to become 'one of the lads'. Wendy describes such a group:

> They brag about who they've got off with, who they want to get off with and things like that. It's just out of order, but they do. We used to go out down the sheds.

> They come to you and say, 'Guess who I've just been with.' Y'know, 'I was with Jimmy.' I mean, we didn't know. She was trendy and had her own mates. She just come round, ponced a fag or something. Then just turned round and said that to us. We didn't want to know about it.

Wendy strongly disapproves of this:

> I mean, say someone would tell their own little group but this girl – she told us – we hadn't got nothing to do with her. Just showing off.

Then there are examples of girls boasting about being on the pill:

> This group I know, certain groups of about seven girls, are on the pill and they really love talking about it. Not sex but that they're on the pill. They say, 'I sort of went out with him and got off with him.' They just do it to impress.

Many girls and boys disapprove of girls who behave in this way. Several girls and boys refer to girls who assimilate characteristics of 'maleness'. Girls are often excluded from the male group and boys who are seen to be too friendly with girls are often called wimps or even poofs. Some boys resent tomboys for subverting natural differences too. As I mentioned in Chapter 2, gender dichotomies require collective activity to maintain them, and although individuals can deviate, their deviance will give rise to disapproval. An example of this is Harry's mixed feelings about Jasmin's tomboyish behaviour, which he found threatening:

> The girls with the big mouths. They keep running me down. Jasmin. She copies all the words I use. In D. and T. (Design and Technology) she always talks to me. She's got the same type of interests. She likes the same type of music.

Harry is aware that Jasmin shares his interests and faces a contradiction in her refusal to adopt the submissive feminine role, and in criticizing him. Such contradictions illustrate the complexity of identity formulation and how feminine and masculine identities are in flux.

Tomboys are more confident than other girls. They are often middle-class, both black and white, but not necessarily so. Many black and white working-class girls are very confident. They do not see themselves as inferior to boys. Tania, a black girl, describes how she goes stealing things with twenty or so boys aged between fifteen and twenty-five years old.

> Sometimes we go into this minicab place. They've got pool and table tennis and all that. Space invaders. When someone's run out of money they just go round the cars. You know the big windows that you wind down? And you've got a little side window. Well they kick that window – it don't make much noise – and put your hand in to open the door, and just get out the speakers. You sell them for around £25 ... Obviously you could get more for radio cassettes than you can for speakers unless you can get good ones like Pioneers. Then you could get £50. Or we'll raid a place where they got a pool table and ping-pong machines.
>
> Q *What do you do with the money?*
>
> Keep it. Let it thaw for about a week, then you go out and buy a kebab or something. You really enjoy yourself and then you buy shoes, clothes or little odds and ends that you need or a trip down the West End ... I know it's wrong, right, to nick from other people. But it's something to do. I've had six bikes within a short period of time ... not one I've bought. It's that bad. If it wasn't for other people pushing me I'd be too scared.
>
> Q *What if you get caught?*
>
> Never been caught. If you get caught the first two or three times nothing happens, right? You get caught about four times and the police really get to know you and they give you a caution. Often there're thirty of us.
>
> Q *Do you think you're different from other girls?*

I was brought up mostly with my brother. I used to just hang around with him, and all down my street were all boys. I was the only girl, so I just sort of act like them because I'm not wanting to stay in the house all the time. If you hit me I'm going to hit you back.

Another term that is used to describe this kind of girl is 'butch'. Chloe, aged fifteen and white, explains to me what it means:

You can be quite butch if you want, it's up to you.

Q *What does butch mean?*

You're quite boyish, thinking about mostly boy things, you know, say you don't want a husband – think they're no good. You get a motor bike 'cos most girls have mopeds . . .

The most successful forms of subversion are collective. One tactic is for girls to brag themselves about their sexual activities. Tania disapproves of this:

She just turned round and said, 'Yeah, we went to his house and he put it in me and we had it off. My mate was sitting in the next room and she didn't even know. Then we thought his mum was back but when we found out she wasn't we went to the bathroom and we did it again.' It's awful isn't it? Bragging that around. How does she know we won't go back and tell? That's out of order.

It does appear that there is a significant change in the confidence of young women to resist the subordinate role and they are beginning to challenge collectively the old stereotypes of masculinity and femininity. Verbal abuse always takes place within a sexual context and its meaning, as with subversion, can be changed by the responses girls make. They are constrained by language but mocking can be a very successful tactic.

Donna Eder (1992) in a study of predominantly white girls in the American Midwest shows how talk is used as a collective process as a way to transform gender relations and can be seen as a form of resistance to traditional female roles with such mocking comments directed at a boy as 'Come over here I'll run your family life.' She illustrates how girls mock many aspects of traditional female behaviour. Teasing often takes the form of goading girls about being sexy or can have a romantic aspect. Girls who are sexy are teased for having dirty minds. It seems to be all right to be sexual, but not too sexual. Boys are also insulted about their sexual inadequacy.

Beverley Skeggs (1991), a British socilogist, describes how students in the group she studied felt able to make regular confrontational stands, which sexualized classroom interaction, in order to embarrass and humiliate male teachers by goading them about the assumed size of their penises:

MANDY Bloody hell, what the heck could you do with that, not much.
THERESE Can't believe he's got kids. With one that size you'd think he'd never be able to get it up.

These comments, according to Beverley Skeggs, successfully challenge the prerogatives of masculine power even if momentarily. Girls refuse to take masculinity seriously. They understand its vulnerabilities: size, performance and potency. These young women are able to use their knowledge of masculinity to subvert the regulatory mechanisms (Skeggs 1991:134).

Attitudes Towards Feminism

Girls who criticize the double standard and boys' behaviour are open to all the ridicule, disdain and anxiety that patriarchy reserves for its critics.[1] They are written off as anti-men, or man-haters, which is ironic in view of the misogyny that they are daily confronted with. Sadly, it is difficult for young women not to be influenced by images of the women's movement as angry, exclusively lesbian, narrow-minded and disturbing.

Veronica, a middle-class girl, when asked what she thought of the women's movement, replied:

> Not good. Most of it. I think some people go too far.
>
> Q *How do you mean?*
>
> I mean they just sort of say, 'Oh, we hate men, men are really the end.' I think that's going too far and that's just being chauvinist yourself about men. But I do agree with things like women should have equal pay and things like that.

Other comments included:

> Anti-men . . . like women on top.
>
> Like stereotyped women. Women who are completely anti-men . . .
>
> I know this sounds as if I'm anti women's lib, but at the moment I think it used to be the man that had the job and the woman who stayed at home and I think it should be like a medium, where whichever one wants to go out apart from at the birth of a child when the woman's the only one who can look after it, but at the rate it's going it'll be the woman who is kicked out whether she likes it or not.

Women's lib can appear to be threatening to girls who fear their territory, the home, may be invaded and they will lose the little space that they have. Feminism stressing autonomy and independence conflicts with the attributes of femininity, and is threatening for girls who are struggling to establish an identity. Some retreat and advocate conventional submissive behaviour. Most girls seem to find the views of feminists very extreme, though what they really mean is that they conflict with conventional subordination. Take these comments:

> It's really bad – women are pushing. It's all extremists . . . I mean women's libbers.
>
> I don't like some people involved in it. Their strong attitudes. They want things that shouldn't be and they want equality.

Sasha, above, rejects the whole idea of equality and is not

even keen on the idea of equal rights, but colludes with inequality, reverting to the age-old distinction between the physical strength of men and women:

> I don't agree with equal jobs for everyone. Anything mental we can do but physical ... To be honest you wouldn't want to be a truck-driver or pull down buildings. Things like furniture removals when you've got to carry heavy loads on your back ... I mean, I think there're a lot of things women couldn't do.

And Anna argues:

> I think that women should always be the housewife. I'm not saying she should always cook, but I think, well they [i.e. the roles of men and women] should be a bit joint, but I definitely think she should do most of it ... It wouldn't hurt if the man Hoovered though ...

Feminism is invariably linked with lesbianism, and lesbian girls are seen as a threat, although few girls even acknowledge knowing one, let alone being lesbian. Fear of seduction by lesbian girls was a constant theme – astonishing in the light of the real harassment that girls experience in their day-to-day life from boys, which often passes as 'natural':

> Maybe we feel threatened by them – so we think to ourselves, 'Oh my God, maybe if they tried to drag me into that thing.'
>
> I think they'd start kind of threatening you, hassling you.

If a close friend came out as a lesbian one girl says:

> I wouldn't talk to her as much as I used to, not because I didn't like her as much but because I'd be threatened by her.

Generally therefore, feminism is regarded negatively and seen as extreme. This may change at university. In a recent study of girls at two universities in the United States, the labels 'libber' and 'feminist' both referred to women involved in or sympathetic to the women's movement, yet one label conveyed a negative valuation of such women and the other a more positive evaluation. Indeed, at one university feminists developed a flamboyant counter-culture (Holland and Eisen-hart 1990). In Britain my impression is that over the last five years the term feminist has become more acceptable.

The Backlash

We can see how threatening feminism is to masculine identity and power and how likely it is to lead to a backlash. This backlash is reported by Susan Faludi to be in full swing in the USA (Faludi 1992), where myths abound: thousands of working women have fled back to the home; feminism's battle has been won; career women destroy themselves, burn out; the 'great emotional depression' for single women; and 'the man shortage', a *Newsweek* story that claimed that a single, college-educated woman of thirty-five was more likely to be killed by a terrorist than get married. Faludi showed that each finding was based on surveys that were later discredited, but their falsity was given little media coverage. In 1986, for instance, bachelors outnumbered unmarried women by 2.5 million in America.

The anti-feminist backlash has been set off not by women's achievement of full equality but by the increased possibility that they might win it. It is a pre-emptive strike that stops women long before they reach the finishing line (Faludi 1992).

In Britain, feminism has been labelled with a list of pejorative terms. Cynthia Cockburn, who undertook a study of the implementation of equal-opportunity policies in four British organizations, was told that women's libbers were harsh, strident, demanding, uptight, aggressive, vociferous, dogmatic, radical, zealots, crusaders, and overly ambitious . . . Feminists bash people over the head with their ideas, they ram things down your throat, take things to ridiculous lengths, niggle about semantics, and, not surprisingly given all this put people's backs up (Cockburn 1991:165). And, of course, they have no sense of humour! Cockburn argues that this reflects an anathematizing of feminism, by which women who declare themselves as feminists lose men's respect. She sees this anti-feminism as a way of policing women's consciousness and preventing the few women who are in positions of authority from furthering women's interests.

In response to similar stereotyping, we have seen teenage girls withdraw from naming themselves feminists lest they be seen as extremists, man-hating lesbians. To argue for the 'construction' of masculinities and femininities involves a clash with all the taken-for-granted 'naturalness' of sexual behaviour. Women who put forward feminist ideas are placed in a contradictory position. To criticize the construction of femininity places one out on a limb, as the threatening usurper of male dominance. The 'slag' construction, as we have seen, is the weapon that can be used to degrade any woman, not just a woman who steps out of line on the acceptable standards of femininity.

The backlash may not be so virulent in Britain because feminism has not gained so much ground. In spite of the rhetoric, there has been no marked change in the distribution of power between the sexes in Britain during the last ten years. Women are still as disadvantaged in terms of education, employment, wealth and power. The 1990 report of the Hansard Society Commission for Parliamentary Reform on 'Women at the Top' documents how in actuality little change has been achieved in women's access to positions of power (Hansard Report 1990). Sex discrimination has hardly been addressed in spite of national and international legislation that should protect the rights of girls and women in education. The Local Education Authorities and the governing bodies of grant-maintained schools are under a general duty to provide facilities for education which are free from sex discrimination, but little progress has been made to achieve this (Section 25 (6) (c) (1) of the Sex Discrimination Act). Though more women are entering higher education than ever before, there is no evidence that the curriculum has shifted dramatically to take gender into account. Between 1975 and 1988 the proportion of women in senior academic posts has scarcely increased from an already derisory number. The proportion of women lecturers, readers and professors has hardly changed over the past half century. Only 16 per cent of university lecturers are women, and a mere 3 per cent of professors. There is evidence too that this is not due to the failure of women to put themselves forward but to the in-built and frequently unconscious biases of appointments panels, which are largely composed of white middle-class men. These men are serviced by poorly paid or unpaid women, not merely at home by their wives, but also at work where cleaners, secretaries and research assistants are overwhelmingly female. Women, on the other hand, who try to combine child-rearing and career are given no help by the institution and only rarely by husbands. It is difficult to explain how higher education can still be guilty of such discrimination on the grounds of race and sex, while maintaining a popular liberal veneer. Alison Utley in the *Times Higher Educational Supplement* described the situation as 'at best an anomaly, at worst a national scandal' (Utley 1990).

In this chapter we have seen how girls adopt different strategies to deal with sexist language. Some of these are more successful than others and some (like feminism) carry the risk of ostracism in the same way other forms of non-conformity do. I have shown how all girls are faced with the difficulties of combating the sexism that is so pervasive throughout society and spend inordinate amounts of energy finding a way to cope with or survive the objectification and subordination that entraps girls. Yet increasingly girls are contesting the sexist discourses and questioning the sexism that a few years ago was so taken for granted.

Notes

1. Simone de Beauvoir described the verbal 'firestorm' she was faced with on the publication of *The Second Sex*:

I received – some signed and some anonymous – epigrams, epistles, satires, admonitions and exhortations addressed to me by, for example, 'some very active members of the First Sex'. Unsatisfied, frigid, priapic, nymphomaniac, lesbian, a hundred times aborted – I was everything, even an unmarried mother. People offered to cure me of my frigidity or to temper my labial appetites; I was promised revelations, in the coarsest terms, but in the name of the true, the good and the beautiful, in the name of health and even of poetry (de Beauvoir 1963).

Bibliography

Ardener, E., 1975, 'Belief and the Problem of Women' in Ardener, S. (ed), *Perceiving Women*, Dent

Beauvoir, S. de, 1963, *Memoirs of a Dutiful Daughter*, translated by James Kirkup

Brah, A., and Minhas, R., 1985, 'Structural Racism and Cultural Difference: Schooling for Asian Girls', in Weiner, G., *Just a Bunch of Girls*, Open University Press

Cameron, D., 1985, *Feminism and Linguistic Theory*, Macmillan

Campbell, A., 1981, *Girl Delinquents*, Blackwell

Cixous, H., 1975, *'Sorties'*, *The Newly Born Woman*, translated by Betsy Wing, University of Minnesota Press, 1986, quoted in Sellers, S., 1991, *Language and Sexual Difference*, Macmillan

Cockburn, C., 1991, *In the Way of Women*, Macmillan

Coward, R., 1992, 'Lash Back in Anger: Have Feminists Fired a War on Women?' in the *Guardian*, 24 March 1992

Daly, M., 1978, *Gyn/Ecology: The Metaphysics of Radical Feminism*, Beacon Books

Datesman, S., and Scarpitti, F., 1977, 'Unequal Protection for Males and Females in Juvenile Court', in Ferdinand, T. N. (ed.), *Juvenile Delinquency in Beverly Hills*, Sage

Eder, D., 1992, 'Girls Talk About Romance and Sexuality', paper given at Alice in Wonderland Conference, Amsterdam, June 1992

el-Saadawi, N., 1988, *Memoirs of a Woman Doctor*, Saqi Books

Evans, G., 1980, 'Those Loud Black Girls', in Spender, D., and Sarah, E. (eds.), *Learning to Lose*, Women's Press

Faludi, S., 1992, *Backlash*, Chatto and Windus

French, M., 1978, *The Women's Room*, André Deutsch

Hansard Society Commission, 1990, Report on Women at the Top, Hansard Society for Parliamentary Government

Holland, D., and Eisenhart, M., 1990, *Educated in Romance: Women, Achievement and College Culture*, University of Chicago Press

hooks, b., 1981, *Ain't I a Woman*, South End Press

hooks, b., 1989, *Talking Back: Thinking Feminist – Thinking Black*, Sheba Feminist Publishers

Irrigaray, L., 1985, *This Sex Which is Not One*, translated by Catherine Porter, Cornell University Press

Jones, C., 1985, 'Sexual Tyranny: Male Violence in a Mixed Secondary School', in Weiner, G. (ed.), *Just a Bunch of Girls*, Open University Press

Kelly, E., 1988, *Surviving Sexual Violence*, Polity

Mahony, P., 1985, *Schools for the Boys? Coeducation Reassessed*, Hutchinson

Sellars, S., 1991, *Language and Sexual Difference*, Macmillan

Skeggs, B., 1991, 'Challenging Masculinity and Using Sexuality', in *British Journal of Sociology of Education*, Vol. 12, No. 2

Spender, D., 1980, *Man Made Language*, Routledge and Kegan Paul

Stafford, A., 1991, *Trying Work*, Edinburgh University Press

Tajfel, H., 1978, *Differentiation between Social Groups: Studies in the Social Psychology of Intergroup Relations*, Academic Press

Utley, A., 1990, 'Direct Action for a Liberal Code', in *The Times Higher Educational Supplement*, 10 Aug.

Walker, S., 1983, 'Gender, Class and Education: A Personal View', in Walker, S., and Barton, L. (eds.), *Gender, Class and Education*

Walkerdine, V., 1990, *Schoolgirl Fictions*, Verso

Weiner, G. (ed.), 1985, *Just a Bunch of Girls*, Open University Press

Chapter 8
Deconstructing Masculinity and Femininity

This book has focused on the way masculine and feminine identities are constituted and reconstituted, developed and resisted in the day-to-day life of adolescent boys and girls. Through the analysis of the terms in which girls and boys talk about their lives, I have shown how they live in very different social worlds. The construction of masculinity and femininity that I have examined, as portrayed to me by what girls and boys have to say about their friendships, schooling, their views of marriage and the future, their attitudes to violence and fighting, their views of sexuality, indicates that girls' day-to-day experience is still subordinate, though many girls have found ways of resisting. I have shown the irrelevance of viewing female adolescence as the development of autonomy and indicated the importance of examining gender relations in order to understand how identities are constituted and reconstituted. I have shown that masculinity and femininity are only meaningful in relation to each other. In order to develop a masculine identity a boy needs to dissociate himself from all that is feminine. He needs to denigrate girls in order to dominate them.

In the introduction I criticized previous models of socialization, which had presented an over-deterministic view of how we develop identities. I suggested that the way masculinity and femininity are constituted changes in different historical periods. A little over a hundred years ago women had no right to education, no right to the custody of their children, no right to keep their earnings if they were married, no right to the vote and few legal rights. Virginia Woolf describes in *A Room of One's Own*, published in 1929, her indignation on discovering that she could not enter the Oxford University library without an escort. This is still the case in many men's clubs, both working-men's and professional clubs. Nor has sexism disappeared at Oxford University. On a recent visit some female students showed me a college rag that had on its front page a league table with girls' names and their sexual contacts. The girls were devastated. Though young women today may not be aware of the resistance the fight for basic human rights aroused from men, they can not be unaware of the inequality they still face.

Transformations in the economy and in the political structure are disrupting traditional notions of masculinity and femininity: the masculine identity of working-class men has been threatened by new technology. The decline in heavy industry, the shift to a service economy and widespread unemployment may have had some effect. Change does not mean that the basic misogyny of the culture as a whole will change. It may even become more entrenched.

Femininity is changing, girls are less romantic and more realistic about what lies in store for them, mocking boys who boast about their sexual prowess. They are critical of the way boys talk about sex, by, for example, going on about how many times they have had it in a day. They are more aware of the double standard, resisting doing all the housework and by and large doing well at school, better than many of the boys. They have more awareness of inequality and the strength of female friendship is gradually gaining recognition. Girls are contesting a passive view of femininity and are increasingly joining the labour force and taking part in public life.

This appears to be particularly true of black girls, who through economic necessity have often had to take on the breadwinner role. Mirza (1992) found that the forms of femininity found among African Caribbean girls were fundamentally different from their white peers. In the black definition, few distinctions were made between male and female abilities and attributes with regard to work and the labour market. She argues that this results in greater equality between black couples where, though they may not necessarily stay together for life, none the less both parties are seen as autonomous individuals in their own right.

On the other hand, the constitution of masculinity has changed little. A few boys I spoke to are aware of issues of equality but the majority, while perhaps not overtly sexist, do little to oppose the sexism around them. Calling girls slags is a way of objectifying them, not recognizing them as people of equal worth. It is also an effective way of controlling female sexuality. The disgust of the female body unless as an object of their desire, epitomized by their views of menstruation, is another form of distancing themselves from everything female. They cannot see the benefits of feminism as their identities have been constituted in opposition to femininity. Sexism should not therefore just be seen as chauvinism. It is deeply ingrained in identity formation, continually endorsed and celebrated by the dominant culture. The mass media, the daily press, pornographic magazines and videos all reinforce the objectifying of women's bodies and celebrate a form of macho, aggressive masculinity. Violence against women is condoned, and the fear of violence constricts the lives of women of all social and ethnic groups.

Jessica Benjamin (1990), an American psychoanalyst, develops Hegel's idea of the master–slave relationship in order to explain relationships of domination and subordination. Domination, she argues, begins with the denial of dependency, from the denial of recognition. In seeking to dominate, the master objectifies the slave but by so doing is unable to communicate with him. Arthur Brittain describes the potentiality of this position for freedom:

The master as subject receives no 'recognition' from the objectified slave. Ironically, therein lies the possibility of the slave's freedom. The slave begins to 'recognize' that it is his or her labour that

transforms the world. The object talks back, rebels and overthrows
the objectifier. The slave becomes the subject of history. In simpler
language the master knows that the slave can never really be absolutely objectified. He has an intuition of the slave's potential to resist.
He fears the slave's resentment and knows that the only way to hold
on to what he possesses is constantly to be on his guard (Brittain
1989:170).

It is the slave who is in touch with reality. The master is
living an illusion, so he can never be free. He does not have
access to the knowledge that the slave has, so he distrusts the
slave. Only the slave can free the master. This can equally be
applied to the way boys dominate girls. Girls are in touch
with reality, with housework, with caring, with the material
world. Boys indulge in illusions, they can be said to live in an
unrealistic dream world. In Anne Stafford's (1991) research
the girls talked about relationships. The boys 'mouth', or
make up stories of sexual conquests, they boast about their
prowess, their bravery: boys with their toys, toys that can be
lethal. A young unemployed British teenager on his way to be
a mercenary in the war in Serbia for pittance pay, when
interviewed on TV said he wanted to find out what it was like
to kill as many people as the Yorkshire Ripper, only legitim-
ately. Films and videos encourage this macho form of masculinity. The ideology of sexuality is dislodged from reality (see
Barrett 1980).

A crucial aspect of the function of verbal sexual abuse is the
denial of dependence. Real communication involves recognizing the other, as existing for herself or himself and not just for
oneself. Otherwise the person may be unable to see that he is
separate from the other. He fails to confront his own dependency. A boy who calls a girl a slag, or describes her in terms of
her body parts – big tits, ginger minge – or in terms of food –
tasty, sweetie – or as a dog or a cow, is denying intersubjectiv-
ity and denying his dependence. She is no more than an
object in his eyes, he is not dependent on her. The way that
heterosexuality is constructed just does not allow for the concep-

tion of female subjectivity, which is why a boy in one of my discussions had not ever considered whether a girl enjoys sex. It is natural for boys to enjoy sex, but not for a girl to. Any girl is always available to the designation slag in any number of ways. The construction of female sexuality involves the construction of a difference between slags and drags: sexuality, presumed to be promiscuous in nature, is not natural for all girls/women but only resides in the slag. A girl who enjoys sex is therefore potentially a slag. It is rarely possible for a woman to be treated as a man's equal intellectually and to be feminine. Men talk of not understanding women, for to understand them would be to reduce their domination, to stop seeing them in terms of their sexuality, as sex objects, but to recognize them as human beings.

Domination therefore denies interrelationships and dependence, not merely in personal relationships but on a world scale. The difficulty of studying autonomy and its related concepts of independence is exacerbated by the present structure of western language. The structure of language is masculine and it distances social realities. The stereotype of woman is very different from the rational autonomous man, the figure who stands for the normal human being. One way forward is to redefine the whole concept of dependence, independence and interdependence.

In making close relationships, dependence is embraced. Vulnerability and need cannot be eliminated. In every close relationship interdependence exists. The conception of the dependent wife and the independent husband is fallacious (see Griffiths 1992). Dependants are not taken to be men and children dependent on a woman for housework and emotional support but women who are dependent on the male wage. Even now when this is not necessarily the case, dependants are usually seen as women. The danger of men denying this dependence is that men no longer recognize their humanity or the humanity of others.

The lack of recognition of female subjectivity has implications far beyond the realm of personal relationships, it has political and cultural implications. Masculine identity is constituted in opposition to everything feminine. It involves a denial of dependence. This leads to the subordination of all aspects of life to the instrumental principles of the public world. The values of private life, the maternal aspects of recognition, nurturance (the recognition of need) and attunement (the recognition of feeling) are seen as threatening. The destruction of these values is a result of the ascendance of male rationality. This conception of independence rests on the depiction of all that is other and alien as the sole guarantee of the subject's freedom.

These constructions of masculinity are endemic to the processes of thought and educational values that inform our educational institutions. Feminist philosophers have linked constructions of masculinity and femininity with processes of thought, and argue that the concept of the individual is really a concept of the male subject (see Gould 1983). Equally, the rationality that reduces the social world to objects of exchange, calculation and control is in effect a male rationality. It is also the rationality that is predominant in the educational system and in the military. It involves a psychic repudiation of femininity, which includes the negation of dependence and mutual recognition, similar to the social banishment of nurturance and intersubjective relatedness to the private world of women and children.

The toll placed on men to live up to these values in the public sphere means that the family is needed as 'a haven in a heartless world', where qualities of emotional support, caring and love are emphasized and where men can recover. Woman took on the 'expressive' role, man the 'instrumental'. Talcott Parsons (1951), an American sociologist, recognized that a modern capitalist society posed problems for stability, which is why the family has been regarded as crucial to maintaining this social stability. This is perhaps why politicians blame the increase in violence among young men on the breakdown of the family and in particular on the increase in the proportion of one-parent families and the absence of male authority. They fail to see that the alienation of these young men arises from the way masculinity is constituted and culturally endorsed. Young men are not encouraged to value family life and child-rearing but led to assume that women will carry on taking the responsibility both for domestic and childcare.

Feminists propose an alternative moral vision that would question the condoning of violence both in the personal and public sphere. To return to Virginia Woolf and the way our educational institutions are geared towards militarism and war, she argued that her male contemporaries were acting as if Mussolini's and Hitler's ideas about how society should be ordered had nothing to do with similar views expressed by clerics in the Church of England or Oxford dons. (The same could be said of the rhetoric about Saddam Hussein in the Gulf war. Education is not immune to the creation of a society that invests more in high tech weaponry than in the skills of negotiation.) She wrote:

Education . . . does not teach people to hate force, but to use it . . . Far from teaching the educated generosity and magnanimity, it makes them on the contrary so anxious to keep their possessions, that 'grandeur and power' of which the poet speaks, in their own hands, that they use not force but much subtler methods than force when they are asked to share them . . . And are not force and possessiveness very closely connected with war? (Woolf 1938:35)

This construction of sexuality which denies women subjectivity and relegates dependence and need to the private sphere of the family has consequences far beyond the interrelationships between men and women.

The implications of gender inequality and the objectification of women are therefore of concern as much to men as to women. Brittain draws attention to the almost exclusive preponderance of men in the military and nuclear establishments, the universities, the multinational corporations, and how they benefit as much as ever from women's reproductive labour. He pessimistically adds that 'Given enough time it is more than likely that our generals, politicians and nuclear scientists will end up destroying us all' (Brittain 1989:198).

Among the major western countries the USA and the UK spend the highest proportion of their national income on the military and have the two slowest-growing economies. Carol Cohn (1987) described how when working for the American nuclear establishment she became aware that the scientists talked in a technical language which was loaded with sexist meaning. It was impossible, she writes, not to notice the ubiquitous weight of gender, both in social relations and in the language of war and militarism, which reflects and shapes the nature of American nuclear strategic projects. By the elaborate use of abstraction and euphemism, the appalling reality of war is forgotten. The talk is of 'clean' bombs and 'clean' language, countervailing attacks rather than incinerating cities, collateral damage rather than human death. The air force does not target people, it targets factories and missile bases. American military dependence was explained as 'irresistible because you get more bang for the buck'. Another lecturer solemnly and scientifically announced 'to disarm is to get rid of all your stuff'. Talk is about erector launchers, soft lay downs, deep penetration and 'releasing 70–80 per cent of our megatonnage in one orgasmic whump' (according to a military adviser to the National Security Council). One professor spoke of India's explosion of the nuclear bomb as 'losing her virginity'. Initiation into the nuclear world involves 'being deflowered', losing one's innocence, knowing sin, all wrapped into one. New Zealand's refusal to allow nuclear-armed or nuclear-powered warships into its ports prompted similar reflections on virginity. The air force maga-zine's advertisements for new weapons rival *Playboy* as a catalogue of men's sexual anxieties and fantasies as Smith illustrated in her description of an air force base at Haywards Heath in Britain (Smith 1989). Feminists have argued that missile envy is one factor behind the build up of nuclear power.

Though some boys in my sample are certainly less openly sexist than others (several talked about the need 'to keep their head down' if they wanted to avoid engaging in sexist banter and the danger of being called a wimp or a poof), the dominance of sexist attitudes so pervasive throughout the culture makes it hard for them not to be affected by such constructions.

In this book I have emphasized the role of language in the construction and perpetuation of women's oppression. The repression of sexuality to the conventional pattern of marriage means that female sexuality has little autonomous expression but is constrained by social station and its duties. The woman becomes the housewife and her virtue comes to consist of the correct performance of the duties of the marital relationship, being a good wife and mother, in which sexual expression is allowed only to the extent of meeting her husband's 'legitimate' sexual needs. If in the private sphere it is woman's duty to keep quiet and be a good wife, in the public sphere her inability to achieve subjectivity closely follows from the way she is defined in terms of her sexuality. She is also seen as responsible for meeting male sexual needs and controlling male violence. Because the male 'rational man' is only possible where his sexual and irrational behaviour can be attributed to woman trouble or other feminine influence, it is obviously impossible, under present circumstances, for men and women to co-exist as equals.

But women are resisting and increasingly leaving unhappy marriages, returning to education and developing subversive strategies. Their economic situation though, unequal in all sorts of ways, is significantly different from what it was twenty years ago. Boys' anxiety and confusion expresses itself in ugly terms. Nor are they encouraged to develop alternative subjectivities by the wider culture. But culture is not an unchanging entity. Men and women make their own culture, in the sense that they are constantly adapting to new circumstances. And it is in men's interests to change and to take on responsibility for, and integrate their sexuality into, their public behaviour. It would mean taking on domestic and child-care responsibilities. It would mean treating women in the public sphere as equals rather than as there on sufferance. The challenging of male and female behaviour may be the source of unhappiness, but it also opens up possibilities for transformation.

Girls see through boys' boasting. They know that boys 'mouth'. They are developing a vocabulary to put men down. They are more realistic. Some are not getting married. And many are determined to be equals with men.

Various explanations have been put forward by feminist writers to explain misogyny. Dinnerstein (1987) argues that men's denigration of women arises from the feelings of vulnerability emanating from the power mothers had over them in early childhood. Concurring with this position, Chodorow (1978) stipulates that only when men take part in childcare will change ensue. But to change the constructions of masculinity and femininity will involve a far more radical change than merely altering the distribution of childcare. It will mean a fundamental shift in our conceptions of masculinity and femininity and their relations to dominant conceptions of rationality and morality.

Bibliography

Barrett, M., 1980, *Women's Oppression Today*
Benjamin, J., 1990, *The Bonds of Love*, Virago
Brittain, A., 1989, *Masculinity and Power*, Basil Blackwell
Chodorow, N., 1978, *The Reproduction of Mothering*, University of California Press
Cohn, C., 1987, 'Sex and Death in the Rational World of Defence Intellectuals', in *Signs*, Vol. 12, no. 4, pp. 687–718
Dinnerstein, D., 1987, *The Rocking of the Cradle and the Ruling of the World*, Women's Press
Gould, C. (ed.), 1983, *Beyond Domination: New Perspectives on Women and Philosophy*, Rowman and Littlefield

Griffiths, M., 1992, 'Autonomy and the Fear of Dependence', in *Women's Studies International Forum*, Vol. 15, No. 3, pp. 351–62

Mirza, H. S., 1992, *Young, Female and Black*, Routledge and Kegan Paul

Parsons, T., 1951, *The Social System*, Chicago Free Press

Smith, J., 1989, *Misogynies*, Faber and Faber

Stafford, A., 1991, *Trying Work*, Edinburgh University Press

Woolf, V., 1929, *A Room of One's Own*, Harcourt

Woolf, V., 1938, *Three Guineas*, Hogarth Press

Index

abortion 11, 189, 190, 211, 221; in USA 190, 204, 216
Abrams, D. 200–201
abuse, verbal 21, 28, 34–49; acceptance of validity 51, 61, 63, 266, 267–8, 277; of boys 33, 39–40, 89–90, 94 (lack of terms for) 7, 31, 32, 39, 210, 262, 276, 310; condoned 181–2, 256–7; denial of dependence 304; effect 49–57; girls police each other by 61, 63, 269; girls' reaction 263; and objectification 20, 304–5; in Parliament 221; and pregnancy 203; sexual slant 28; subversion 285–93; and suicide 250; victim blamed 252–3; *see also* poof; slag
adolescence 29, 63; autonomy 12, 13, 15–17, 301, 305; identity 5, 14, 16–17, 146, 303
Afro-Caribbeans 122, 195, 285–6; and education 163–4, 165–6; women's status 165–6, 302–3
AIDS 94, 191–2, 200, 216, 221; and condom use 47, 192, 198, 262; education on 187–8, 196, 198, 203
Allport, Gordon 58
anger 62, 227–8, 293
anorexia 85, 209, 227, 250, 262

anxiety 209, 233–4, 309
appearance: and career 168; girls' fights over 96–7; and identity 264–5; as provocative 31, 228–9, 231–2; and racism 60–61; and reputation 15–16, 31, 36, 42–4, 46, 50, 57, 61, 63
Ardener, E. and S. 286–7
Arnot, M. 33, 64, 157
Asians: diversity 57; education 122, 164–5, 166; employment 57–8, 122; family 33, 57, 82, 94; friendships 93; *izzat* 33, 57, 94; marriage 122, 138–9; and racism 33, 285; religion 57; reputation 17, 32–3, 46; sex education 210; women's isolation 70, 142
attachment 27, 36, 52; *see also* steady relationship
Australia 57, 182, 201, 202, 217, 218, 233–4
autonomy: adolescence and 12, 13, 15–17, 301, 305; and boys' moral judgements 249; feminism and 15, 294; friendships imply 67; loss in steady relationship 29, 63; reformulation 24, 305–6; /self-sacrifice contrast 262; *see also* independence
avoidance strategies 24, 272–5

marriage – *contd*

failure rate 190; Asian 122, 138–9; boys' views 107, 129, 137–43; and career 125–7; for children's sake 105, 106, 124, 129–34; decline in teenage 189–90; education and stress 101; equality and inequality 100–101, 106, 107, 118, 120–21, 127–8, 129, 138–9, 140, 144–5, 309; essentialist idea 155–6, 180; expectation/actuality gap 133; girls' views of 22, 106–7, 114–34; 'having your life' before 106–7, 114, 118, 125, 127, 130, 131; as inevitable 106, 115–16, 124–5, 137, 143; integration into husband's networks and interests 99, 100–101, 105; isolation in 119, 197; love and 107–13; money distribution 118–19, 142–3; postponement 106, 122, 125–7, 137–8, 162; and race 128; and reputation 124–5; 'right man', finding of 106, 121, 124, 127–9; *see also under* employment; housework; realism; sexuality; unemployment; violence; virginity

Marshall, Jane 155

masculinity: deconstructing 301–11; deviance from norm 88; and economic change 146, 257, 309; and education 23, 153, 180–82, 306; and emotions 159, 210, 250–51; hegemonic 95, 210, 287; and language 21, 286, 305; media image 3, 303; militarism 307–8; new forms 105–6, 177,

301–11; and public sphere 245–6, 264–5, 306; and rationality 151, 306; social construction 180–82; tomboys assimilated to 275, 290; work as basis 2, 3, 14, 227, 236, 238, 302; *see also* vulnerability *and under* femininity; race; sexuality; violence

master-slave relationship 303–4

maturity 12

media 3, 237, 303; depiction of body 16, 32, 141, 211–12; *see also* films; magazines; television

medicine 284–5

menstrual extraction 190

menstruation 188, 207–10, 247, 261; boys' attitudes 207–8, 209–10, 233, 303; taboo 207–8, 209, 211, 214–15, 265

Meredith, Philip 220

middle class 118, 129–30, 176; and education 126, 157, 161, 174, 177–8

Mies, M. 12

militarism *see* war

miners' strike 101

misogyny 232–3

Modleski, Tania 113

money 81, 118–19, 142–3, 174, 245, 297

Moore, Suzanne 14

morality 1, 24, 246–9, 310

Morrison, Toni 84

mothers and motherhood 94, 101, 133, 145–6, 262, 310

music, popular 1, 86–7, 95; *see also* pop stars

muted group, women as 286–7

Naber, Pauline 100

READ MORE IN PENGUIN

In every corner of the world, on every subject under the sun, Penguin represents quality and variety – the very best in publishing today.

For complete information about books available from Penguin – including Puffins, Penguin Classics and Arkana – and how to order them, write to us at the appropriate address below. Please note that for copyright reasons the selection of books varies from country to country.

In the United Kingdom: Please write to *Dept. JC, Penguin Books Ltd, FREEPOST, West Drayton, Middlesex UB7 OBR*

If you have any difficulty in obtaining a title, please send your order with the correct money, plus ten per cent for postage and packaging, to *PO Box No. 11, West Drayton, Middlesex UB7 OBR*

In the United States: Please write to *Penguin USA Inc., 375 Hudson Street, New York, NY 10014*

In Canada: Please write to *Penguin Books Canada Ltd, 10 Alcorn Avenue, Suite 300, Toronto, Ontario M4V 3B2*

In Australia: Please write to *Penguin Books Australia Ltd, 487 Maroondah Highway, Ringwood, Victoria 3134*

In New Zealand: Please write to *Penguin Books (NZ) Ltd, 182–190 Wairau Road, Private Bag, Takapuna, Auckland 9*

In India: Please write to *Penguin Books India Pvt Ltd, 706 Eros Apartments, 56 Nehru Place, New Delhi 110 019*

In the Netherlands: Please write to *Penguin Books Netherlands B.V., Keizersgracht 231 NL–1016 DV Amsterdam*

In Germany: Please write to *Penguin Books Deutschland GmbH, Friedrichstrasse 10–12, W–6000 Frankfurt/Main 1*

In Spain: Please write to *Penguin Books S. A., C. San Bernardo 117–6° E–28015 Madrid*

In Italy: Please write to *Penguin Italia s.r.l., Via Felice Casati 20, I–20124 Milano*

In France: Please write to *Penguin France S. A., 17 rue Lejeune, F–31000 Toulouse*

In Japan: Please write to *Penguin Books Japan, Ishikiribashi Building, 2–5–4, Suido, Tokyo 112*

In Greece: Please write to *Penguin Hellas Ltd, Dimocritou 3, GR–106 71 Athens*

In South Africa: Please write to *Longman Penguin Southern Africa (Pty) Ltd, Private Bag X08, Bertsham 2013*